Miracles For Soul Finders

The Mirror Calls For The Unexpected

RITA HARRISON

Published By
BHUTATA INK 2019
www.bhutata.ink

"Copyright © 2019 by Rita Harrison All rights reserved. Except as permitted under the U.S. Copyright Act of 1976, no part of this publication may be reproduced, distributed, or transmitted in any form or by any means, or stored in a database or retrieval system, without the prior written permission of the publisher."

ISBN: 9781718130272

DEDICATION

I dedicate this book to all who wish to take their health and their lives into their own hands and create the unexpected

ACKNOWLEDGMENTS

I want to thank my husband, Paul, for his faith in me, and for helping me to translate the original German version of this book from German, to Germ-Lish, to English.

Thanks to our dear friends Sandra Gabriele and Cristy Murray who helped us in translating and editing this book.

Mahalo to the island of Kaua'i for providing the precious insights and supporting people in my life.

I also want to thank my clients and training participants in Germany, Austria, Canada, England and USA for sharing their lives with me and for allowing me to use their stories so that other people can benefit from their insights as well.

I thank my father, Hans Straub, for guiding me ever since and for giving me the gift to experience a "stateless" and international life. -R.H.

CONTENTS

Dedication
Acknowledgements i
Contents ii

Preface: Or, Something Like It, Anyway 1

The Power Of Being Conscious Miracleness
1   Sometimes Heaven Begins In Hell   5

The Source Of Miracles
2   The Power That Creates Is The Power That Destroys   11
3   The Power Of The Magical Moment   14
4   The Power of Decision   18
5   Focus of Attention: Friend or Foe?   22
6   Short Term Longevity Or Long Term Shortevity?   26
7   The "W" Questions: When is WHY important?   28
8   Passive Believers vs. Active Faith Builders   31
9   The "How" Will Show Up   34
10   The Reward: Subconscious Sustenance   37

The Six Levels Of Being Consciously Miraculous
11   The Miracle of the Six   40
12   The Six Levels Mirrored in Your Decisions   44

Our Bodyhouse: The Constant Place For Miracles
13   Our Body is a Perfect Survival Expert   49
14   Spring Cleaning As A Miracle   53

E-Motion-Ergy
15   Everything Is Energy   58
16   Go As Deep as it Takes   62
17   Riding The Light-Waves   66

A Mentastic World

18	Activating Miraculous Intelligence	69
19	The Power of Conviction	73
20	The Mind: "A Glimmer that Gives The Body A Soul"	75
21	Lack mentality… It's All the Rage!	79
22	Be smart when you're intelligent!	83
23	The Power of Intention	88
24	Made in …Me	92

Unraveling Entanglements

25	The Truth Heals in the Depths	94
26	You Are Also a Product of Your Environment	99

The Miracle Of The Group/Family

27	Group Consciousness: Miracle or Mayhem?	106
28	Making History	109

No Miracles Without Soul

29	Look Who's Talking	114
30	The Camel May Not Have Gone Through the Eye of the Needle Yet…	117
31	Life Purpose: Soul Championship in the Body Olympics	120
32	In This World, But Not Of It…	125

Outside Of Time And Space

33	Communicating with the Whales	128

The Last Words

34	Conclusion	132

About The Author   135

PREFACE
Or, Something Like It, Anyway

Drumbeats...
Let me talk to you as if I were talking to both you and your inner child. Where these two parts of you meet is the place where Conscious MiracleNess happens... where you get access to something unexpected inside you. The Inner child might provide the miracles and the grownup consciousness makes them happen. In this book, you are invited to understand yourself in a way that supports the ongoing creation of miracles, even in situations where you (your grownup self) may have decided no miracle can live.

How does that happen? It happens because the inner child and grownup you work in synergy, finally on the same team, working toward the same purpose. How does this book provide that foundation? By introducing you, the reader, to a totally reworked way of looking at yourself and how you can affect life. By listening to the natural inner wisdom that comes up when you are open... you can then become consciously aware of how miraculous you are.

This book is for everybody who does not yet believe, 100%, that they are capable of being something exceptional... or even astonishing. For everybody who has doubts that they can express their miraculousness.

It is for everybody who tends to trust that somebody else has this gift but not they themselves.

Accordingly, this book is for everybody who longs to radiate Light but, so far, has kept his or her light under a bushel. It's for everybody who wants to be happy, healthy, and fulfilled. It's for everybody who feels the value of feeling freedom and easiness.

This book is for everybody who already believes in their own miraculousness, but may not know how to live it, to manifest it in their every day lives. For those who catch themselves creating explanations for why it isn't possible to live this way, but no longer believe their own explanations.

This book is for the doubters and skeptic, the ones who know that miracles do happen, but hold that separate from their participation. This writing wants to show you that More Miracles actually are the natural consequence of your inner and outer attitudes. When one always waits for miracles to occur without actively participating, ... you can forget it. I invite you now to explore the possibility that You Are the one who creates the exceptional; I invite you to realize your part so you can do it over and over again.

This book is for everybody who has noticed the craziness that's out there, and has made a decision to step out of it, and to step into his or her own inner truth.

- How would you describe yourself?
- To which of these categories do you belong?

Because there are already so many books about this, I want to present this book to you in a totally different way... I will present this from YOUR point of view, and I will get you to help.

WHAT?!?!?! How is it possible that I write a book from your point of view?!?!?!

By inviting you to access your truth, your real and true story, which wants to come out and fully be lived. To access everything that expresses who you really are. So. If you are interested in how you can Miracularize yourself on all levels by allowing yourself to live the Conscious MiracleNess you already are, then you are reading the right book. While you are reading it, I will invite you to answer certain questions.

Why? Because answering these questions makes the difference between just reading a book, and traveling together on a journey. Of course, you don't have to do it this way. You always have the choice. Maybe this will be just another book you read, as opposed to creating a space for making your own history. That's okay as well. Just remember, answering the questions is the key to truly having experiences that change your consciousness and actions.

If you do decide to answer the questions, you don't have to put yourself under pressure to be as genius as possible, or to meet programmed expectations from outside. The purpose of these questions is to allow you to engage with yourself. They shift your focus inside. They make room in which you can experience the truth – that when you focus within, your answers can only be right. Failure will be replaced by success, and you will come to realize that failure itself is a programmed illusion of the past.

So. Where are you right now, in your book of life?

Suppose you used your inherent ability to create outstanding experiences in your life…

- Where would you like to be at the end of the book?
- How would that change your life?
- What do you think would happen next?
- How would that be for you?

Not every question must be answered.
Sometimes, simply to ask the question is enough. It engages your subconscious, and then, even before the answer is known, change happens.

1

The Power Of Being Conscious Miracleness
SOMETIMES HEAVEN BEGINS IN HELL

I am in hell. In the middle of chaos. I feel confused and desperate. Almost no money. Almost no friends. Almost no family. My whole life seems to be falling apart, a deep dark chasm is opening up beneath me. I look into the depths and I fall... and fall, and fall, and fall. And then I land.

Land?! On what?

It feels like standing on confusion. But when I look more closely, it turns out it's a scream. A scream?

Yes. A scream...

I am screaming for a miracle. "I NEED A MIRACLE!!" I cry myself to sleep, and I dream. And in my dream I hear, "The miracle you are looking for Is You.".

Yes. Of course. This is what people always hear. So now what? I am too tired... too disappointed... too ... to make sense of it. Maybe other people can make sense of it, other people in other situations, but not me. What happened was too much. Easy for you to say, but you have no idea how hard this is!!!

With whom am I arguing? Who is it that I'm trying to convince of my helplessness? Of the heaviness of my destiny? Who is it that I am trying to push away, so that I can dig my heels in deeper to the programs of my past and the personalized collective victim consciousness.

It answers back. "It is easier for a camel to slip through the eye of the needle than for a rich man to reach heaven." ... whatever that means.

All of a sudden it becomes clear to me that I am like the camel, standing before the eye of the needle. I recognize as well that I am the rich man too busy complaining to mobilize the power inside me. I could climb up the rope this noose around my neck is hanging from to reach heaven, the Unexpected.

But this is the hard way! It would be easier to moan, to suffer, and to stay in hell. There, I would be one of many. Who would notice among all the other moans? In this place, where everybody walks like each other, and talks like each other, and acts like each other, this is just normal.

If normal could have brought me any further, I wouldn't be here, where I am now.

Huh. Ok. That's true. Perhaps it is time to try something else. And in this quiet recognition, I wake up, now free of the self-talk.

So you are there, seemingly at a point in the road where only stop signs are around you. This book gives you the tools to bustle up the road itself that you stand on and turn this seeming nothingness into something... something miraculous.

We must have a true idea of who is standing on the road in order to build. The gateway to the miracles is in this understanding. Luckily, we need not look far... this is about inside... the person... the mirror of the Unexpected inside you.

This is a reflection of who you really are and it's not new... you will realize as you read this that you know it already. You are Conscious MiracleNess!

Do you need proof? Here it is: you will feel the familiarity of these ideas as you read. You may even catch yourself exclaiming aloud.

If not, you won't have any idea what we are talking about.

So. Who are you, really? Well, let us look at the body. You are, really, a collection of cells. Each cell is specialized and performing a perfect function – to be the blood, to be the liver, to be the brain... Each cell is always in communication with the others, fluidly, rhythmically, some times even faster than light. When your body wants to send you a message, it can only use what is there... it can give you neurological messages, such as pain or comfort, or sensory messages. When the body sends messages by using these specific methods, while you might think, "Oh, what's wrong with me?" the body is actually saying, "Oh, there's nothing wrong... I am just using my self healing power, telling you what's going on so you will take care of me on time and do something about it."

So. Who else are you really? Well, you are someone who experiences emotions. They are there all the time. Sometimes we interpret them as positive, sometimes negative, but they are always there. What are they, really? Think how you feel when you are experiencing positive emotion. You are like a surfer, gliding along on your surfboard, up on top of the open wave. This comes naturally. So now what of the negative emotions? To use their power, you do the same – you feel them, and use them as direction from yourself – they are like indicators when course corrections are necessary. Your emotions tell you, "I am here to help you navigate through all kinds of waters."

So. Who else are you really? As Albert Einstein said, everything is energy. So you are, as well! As humans, we notice this in terms like, "I have no energy for this." Or "I am exhausted." Or "I feel so energized." Or, "I just don't like that guy's vibe." Or, "We are on the same wavelength." Your energy is another messenger, helping you find where you are synchronized with something, and where you are not.

So. Who else are you really? René Descartes, the French Philosopher, Mathematician and writer, said, "I think, therefore I am." And we know this... we are thinking all the time! Thought comes naturally; we are professional thinkers. Thoughts are like the geyser, which flows into our words, which flow into our deeds. At the same time, they inform the filters through which we perceive what's happening around us. This mental level gives us the experience of "I know." Or "I understand." It is also the mechanism that allows us to forget things that do not serve us, or put away things that are over. The mind encourages us, "Think about it. Say it. This has to be done." And in other cases, it says, "Forget that. It is of no use to you now."

So. Who else are you really? Consider yourself as a piece of a puzzle. In order to feel whole, you need the rest of the pieces, and they need you the same way! You are also a being in relationship, no matter what. Unless you are Adam (or Eve), for sure, you landed on this earth as a son or daughter – as part of a larger whole. That Whole talks to you as well, "You are part of the fisherman's net. If the rest of the net falls into the ocean, the currents will affect you. Even if you don't see the ocean, you will feel its pull." It shows you how you interact, even with things you don't directly experience, because you are part of the net. This net, then, also is a messenger – if you are feeling a pull, perhaps you have to straighten your place in the whole, or retie some of the cords between you and the people you are in relationship with.

So. Who else are you really? You are the I Am presence. An eternal essence, expansive and rising. A peaceful peace. The source of these messages that we've been seeing evidenced in the other parts of being human.

The sense of purpose, the awareness that constantly puts your feet on the stairway to heaven, which is the journey of the soul. The soul says, "Everything is going to be okay. We'll be alright. I can see the road ahead, and I am always here, always talking to you."... And sometimes, it says, "Where the hell are YOU?"

So. Who else are you really? You are a messenger yourself and the one who is receiving the messages – both sender and receiver at once. This is another aspect of human existence: right now, right here, there is a system of information exchange in place that happens unlimited by time and space. This is intuition; nonverbal communication, silent Knowing. There is a communication between all of us, just as there is between your cells. As a messenger, you are holding a key for others, and they hold a key for you. A key to unlock the doors. We use the keys, and the light goes on. For example, you think of someone, and they call. Or you find out they have been thinking of you as well. Or you wish for something to happen in your life, and, Whoosh!, there it is!

Where is their support for this, in our physical world? Deep inside every one of us: in our DNA.

The scientific understanding of our DNA, at this moment in history, is undergoing a revolutionary change. In 1990, a group of Russian and American scientists led by a Microbiologist called Dr. Pjotr Garjajev found that rather than being a fixed set of instructions of our physicality, our DNA actually changes continuously throughout our lives. Garjajev and his colleagues learned that our DNA actually sends, receives, and saves information outside of time and space, and that this is based upon our experiences as we live our lives. The scientists use the metaphor of the computer chip – that we are like that chip, constantly engaged in a reprogramming process.

Does this sound fantastic? That right now, the DNA, which is within each of your trillions of cells, is moving light-based   information   around   the   universe?

...Remember, once we thought the earth was flat...

So. Who are you, really?

You are:
- Consciousness
- A Miracle
- Miraculous
- ConsciousMiraculousNess

So now, by allowing yourself this totally fresh, more complete understanding of who you are, you get access to your inherent power to use these miraculous tools to create the unexpected... to surprise yourself... and to enjoy hidden resources (that were always there) that are ready to be lived. The delights can unfold in all kinds of ways – in your health, in your relationships, your creativity, motivations, visions, and decisions.

What happens inside you while you read this?
What if you allowed yourself just a little to step into this kind of view of who you really are? What would be different then? Who else would notice this difference? And how would it influence your every day life?

What if you wanted to surprise yourself and live the unexpected already in certain parts of your life?

How would that look?

2

The Source Of Miracles
THE POWER THAT CREATES IS THE POWER THAT DESTROYS

I believe that everything has a source.

Imagine a spring. The spring becomes the creek and the creek becomes the river and the river flows into the ocean.

This can be likened to constructive and destructive energy within you. If a certain amount of constructive or destructive energy flows long enough, this shapes the inner landscape, and that inner landscape is then mirrored in the outer. We find this in us constantly showing up in our thoughts, feelings, energy levels, bodies, relationships, souls and all parts of our everyday lives. Depending on where you place yourself in relation to the spring, you experience either inspiration or destruction - both important forces. The question is where would you have to position yourself so that you experience a balance of these powers?

I am convinced that there is no fixed place, but, rather, a dynamic movement in which you approach one, then the other, and back again, like a flow in the eternal movement of the water of every life, every death, and every rebirth.

- How do you see it?
- Why is this important?

Both powers exist within each one of us: the constructive, creative power, and the destructive. Nature destroys itself automatically when there is no energy that works against it. For example, if we don't eat, we starve… so we decide to eat. When we don't choose the constructive force, the destructive comes up automatically. This can go even further: when we are in the middle of a destructive phase, we are in danger of forgetting the creative force completely. We can allow the creek of destructive energy to become a river, which still becomes the ocean, but now it's an ocean of destructiveness. The point of change is an active process. It needs energy. To just let it go along is a passive process, and although it might draw energy, it often seems easier than shifting. And the river flows, and the ocean fills, destructive source to destructive outcome.

So when you wish to stop the flow of the destructive river, then you must do something.

- Anything!
- Anything that's possible!
- Not just go with the flow!

When you achieve focus on the creative power, to use it, then real miracles can take place.

- How can you remind yourself of the creative power inside you, while the destructive energy still has the lead?
- Where would you look first for the light, the creative force, in order to find it?
- What would you do with this energy when you've found it?
- What would change by using it?

The art of remembering the light when it is dark creates a distinctive difference in your life. Yes, it even separates the wheat from the chaff and gives you the power to be able to benefit from every so-called negative situation. Your wellbeing becomes more and more independent of outside circumstance.

You don't need to be enlightened to practice enlightenment. Training and knowledge can also help you on your way.

Suppose you were to give yourself the permission to stay in the flow between the rivers of destruction and creation:

- What would happen?
- What would you like the destructive force to remove from your life in order to feel better?
- What would you expect the creative force to give you so that you feel good?

3
The Source Of Miracles
THE POWER OF
THE MAGICAL MOMENT

From my life: It's a hot summer in Germany in August 1983. Usually it's never too hot for me, but this year, it is different.

An exceptional situation...

I sit beside the deathbed of my beloved father. The vision before me, my father struggling with his Breath, the color draining from his face, his life force slipping away. We haven't much time left. My stomach is clenched and I feel frozen and helpless.

Just before he leaves his body completely, his consciousness clears and we share an intense moment that will change my life from that moment forward and all my decisions. At that moment, I was not aware of the breadth of the effect this minute would have on my life. Years later, I understood the depth of the gift that Life gave us in that moment of dying, the power of that magical moment... and again, destruction and creation, hand in hand.

- What does the power of the magical moment mean for you?
- What do you think it is?

For me, it is the following: I am looking at my father breathing heavily, wishing for his release and relief. I am very attached to him, and haven't wanted him to go. But just in that moment, I let go; I wouldn't hold him back anymore, and I realized that I could handle the situation better when I hold tight to something else instead of him. Everything seems to be so intense, so immense, and existential. I understand for the first time that the experience of dying connects me with the natural force of life and that it's all about who I am and what I need; where the others are and what they need, in order to be really happy and fulfilled. In this moment I hear myself talking to my father. "I will learn and study without quitting, until I have found answers enough to help other people."

I give my father a promise that he didn't ask me for. Actually, I give myself a promise, because this promise gives me something to hold onto in this moment. I felt that my father, my previous support, was being taken away. My father is nodding at me. I feel myself so intensely that I recognize my life purpose in the depth of my soul. This means I want to contribute to the decrease of suffering and the increase of joy. By doing that, everybody is cared for automatically. I am cared for and the others are cared for at the same time.

Now how would I do that?

As the eighteen year old I was at that moment I had no clue. But the decision had already begun to influence me. And I realized for the first time that I'm diving for the pearls of light in the darkness. Those bits of light had me say and do things I never dreamt of. I used to be programmed with shyness, shame, unworthiness, and the struggle to survive. And even though I stayed there for a long while, I found my life purpose through that magical moment.

This creates a place for my truth: I find myself by helping others to find themselves. And because we are connected to each other, it doesn't make a difference on whose behalf we come together; both benefit from the answers as long as they are sourced in the deepest truth.

- When did you have your magical moment?
- What did it invite you to discover about yourself?
- What decisions did you make in that moment?
- How did they change your life?
- How can you still draw power out of the intensity of that moment?

Today, I know, by giving my father a promise, I gave myself, unintentionally but sustainably, a kick in the butt. This, this kick in the butt has ensured my sticking to my decisions to this day.

My conscious is constantly reminding me: "There's no going back now, babe. Your best is the least I'll accept. You gave your word and it's golden."

I keep this in the back of my head, in my heart… and this exactly gave, and still gives me, power – the power of the magical moment.

The trick is to tell somebody. Somebody that you don't want to disappoint, just in case you find out that you want to back out of your promise – escape from your own power.

And in addition to that, we have the following. At that time of my life, my own sense of self worth was not high enough that making the promise to ME would have mattered… so instead I used a trick: I gave it to someone to whom I attached the greatest value: my Papa.

Another element that reinforced the power of that moment was that I knew my father believed in me, so much more than I could believe in me. He was nodding, encouraging me, "Yes, girl, go for it" … like a blessing. Even when I didn't believe I could do it.

- Which kind of promise would do you and your life good?
- To whom would you make this promise in order to give yourself a kick in the butt?
- How would that change your life?
- Which kind of blessing would you need to make it real?
- When are you going to take your reward?

4
The Source Of Miracles
THE POWER OF DECISION

Cross your heart. Do you also think sometimes that it would be easier to make your wishes come true if you had certain other conditions… for example, more money, time, or self-confidence? Do you? Be honest with yourself. Do you catch yourself falling into programmed helplessness instead of creating for yourself the conditions for fulfillment?

Do you hear yourself saying, "Oh, that's not possible, because…" when an opportunity comes up that could change your currant situation?

Then this chapter is the right place to be.

Some questions that we ask when we are feeling sorry for ourselves are conditioned and worthless. Yes. You read that right. They are worthless, but we ask them anyway.

An example of worthless question is, "What did I do wrong?" The answers that follow can only be negative. Ok. Sometimes you need to know these things. But does this kind of knowledge really make a difference? I doubt it.

So, why do we ask questions that don't make a difference?

Maybe it's out of habit or custom. Or maybe it's because we don't have any better questions to ask at that moment in time.

So, let's fix this situation right now!

I give you a few alternative questions to ask instead so you can condition yourself anew and replace the old habitual questions. As you may, or may not remember from the last chapter, we only let go of old habits when we have something better to replace them with.

Let's suppose you could have some influence on a currant situation as it is now:

- What would you do differently than you did before?
- How would you start?
- What would be your very first step?
- What would be the next step?
- …And then?

What would you expect it to change?

- In you?
- For you?
- For your world?
- For the people around you?

Take your time to answer the questions before you read on.

Anthony "Tony" Robbins, an American self-help author and success coach, tells us in one of his publications that people who are successful in spite of being subjected to appalling conditions very often distinguish themselves by making different decisions than those who moan.

What also is needed is that you make a new contract with yourself, which can be difficult for most of us. The contract in question is that you are allowed to make mistakes. When you don't dare to make mistakes, then it might be that you don't dare to do anything at all. Dissatisfaction, envy, and negativity feed on this state of affairs.

Maybe your focus of attention is on the outside rather than on the inside, which can lead to a loss of power and energy, instead of using your energy from the inside out for positive effect.

Not to make a decision at all may seem better for most of us.

We often don't see that not deciding is a decision as well with the side effect of giving away our power instead of using it.

We react instead of acting.

Every form of decision determines the consequences there of.

So, it is wise to face the consequences before they happen.

Suppose you are able to make a conscious decision:

- What decision would you like to make so that your wishes would come true?
- How would you show your environment that you have made this decision?
- Which consequences would this decision produce?
- For you?
- For other people who are involved?
- Which kind of mistakes would you allow yourself to make eventually?

At this point I would like you to redefine in your vocabulary the meaning of the word 'mistake'.

In actuality, mistakes are not mistakes!

They are experiences that help us find out which decisions are good and which decisions are bad, all of which helps us to make new and better decisions as we move through life.

- How does this feel to you?

5
The Source Of Miracles
FOCUS OF ATTENTION: FRIEND OR FOE?

Your focus of attention determines where your energy goes. It determines what you perceive, and how you perceive it. It acts like a filter, and through it, you recognize some things as the truth, but see others not at all. Sometimes even positive things, according to your own filter, can hide from you, like health within a story of illness, or a hidden talent when you feel you actually failed.

This focus determines how you feel, your ability to receive gifts from life, and how you proceed in life. It determines whether you experience having a lot of energy and motivation or little.

And so on…

Your upbringing, education, habits, etc. have a big influence on your focus of attention.

Here is an example:
In times of financial difficulty, most people only think about money and focus on "There is not enough" all the time. "How can I keep my head above water?" determines their daily decisions.

Every decision has a consequence, every river flows from its source. In this example the focus of attention leads to only being able to hold your head above water, no more, no less. This kind of source creates a river of 'just surviving'.

If they had put their focus on what they really wanted and what gave them motivation and power, yes, maybe even enthusiasm and energy, then they would have experienced something completely different, like perhaps learning a totally new job, or adjusting their ideas about how they earn money, to be more in line with the actual situation.

A lot of people have become rich in times of economic depression because they had a flash of inspiration that fit the needs of the times.

Flexibility helped them to keep their focus on possibilities and not on lack of the times!

Suppose you could be more flexible in a situation?

- Where would your focus of attention be?
- Would it be on lack? Or on new possibilities and the things you really want?

How would that influence your actions?

- What would you have to focus on in order to gain more motivation, power, and drive to move forward?
- How would you realize that you are on the right track?
- How would you recognize where your focus of attention is?

My answer would be: Observe yourself!

Here, it might be useful to slip out of your own self, and to look at you from above, or from outside, from a meta level. An inner, higher seat that you sit on, which gives you a broader perspective.

I invite you to be nosy.

Look at yourself as someone fascinating, go out of your way to find the astonishing you!
Choose to look at the whole thing with humor… to season the experience with a smile on your face… maybe even assuming the role of the Omnipotent Narrator… "Aaah! Look at Me! Look at what I'm doing now! How interesting!"

- What do you think you need to change – to really change – your focus?

May I make a suggestion? Remind yourself to use your inherent discipline to direct your focus consciously to where it serves you best.

Pardon?

What do you mean you have no discipline??? *Ha ha ha…I'm not buying that!*

What do you think you have been using that has kept you in your moaner, victim, that's-just-the-way-it-is mode for such a long time?
Yes, it's there: Discipline!!!
The only question is now:

- How do you want to use it?
- For yourself?
- Or against yourself?

Suppose you decided to use it for yourself…

- What would you do?

6
The Source Of Miracles
SHORT TERM LONGEVITY OR LONG TERM SHORTEVITY?

The proof is in the pudding.

Wanda came into my practice. She suffered from chronic back pain, problems with the shoulders, and couldn't sleep at night.

She said that she had been referred to me long ago, but had limited insurance, so she first went to all the other places that were covered by her insurance plan... but didn't find the relief she was looking for.

We found out that her problems came from her jaw and a twisted pelvis. Furthermore we discovered that since the birth of her daughter, she had never found her way back to her natural sleeping rhythm.

After two sessions of treating the root causes of her problems and not just the symptoms, she described an immense improvement.

What was at play here?

Wanda did what many of us do: She was saving money in the wrong places!

She decided to pursue short-term benefit by saving

money, but in the long run she paid more… she paid with her health and her quality of life. In addition, she would have been able to return to work earlier if she had regained her health sooner. The net effect is that altogether she had even lost money because she didn't spend money at the right time.

- What short-term price would you have to pay to achieve what you really want in the long term?
- Which short-term disadvantages would you have to consider now?
- What long-term rewards await you if you acted right now?
- What exactly is it that you would do if you were to act right now?

Take your time to answer the questions with as many details as you can. (By the way, this advice is appropriate for all the answers.)

Even though you may not put everything into action in exactly the way you picture it, but simply by using your imagination and playing with the solutions in your mind, research has shown that you start to reprogram your nervous system, helping you move in the desired direction.

Be aware that in order to get there:

- The decision always has to come first!

Don't put yourself under pressure. Sometimes you may not be able to answer the questions. In those cases, know that simply asking begins the process of change. It might even be that the solution comes after you have stopped thinking about it.

7

The Source Of Miracles
THE "W" QUESTIONS:
WHEN IS WHY IMPORTANT?

Is this familiar?
You're not feeling well or things are not going as you wish. You ask yourself *why* do I feel how I feel? Why aren't things working? Why do I feel so bad? Why is this happening again?

In my 25 years of experience in private practice and seminars, I realize that it sometimes might serve to know the answers to these questions. But that doesn't necessarily mean that they will help you to move on. A lot of people even allow the answers they find to become a reason for NonProgress.

We are all accustomed to asking these W questions and do it habitually. I am not talking about eliminating something that comes so naturally. I propose that the habit can be far more effective if we adjust the content, which I mentioned already in the chapter about the power of decisions.

Instead of asking 'Why' questions that focus on the negative things, or create judgment that leaves you weak, we can turn the questions around and direct them toward empowering, creative, uplifting focus.

Here is an example:

- Why would I like to achieve this goal?

Followed by other powerful 'W' questions:

- What am I expecting afterwards?
- Which elements of personal growth do I expect?
- What would I do differently if I knew that I could not fail?

Notice the power of adding 'I' to the equation.

Structured this way, the answers to the "W" questions connect you to your own motivating power. And this motivating power is the driving force behind success. The more of this power you are in touch with, the better. So fill yourself with this supercharging fuel by contemplating exactly "why do I want" to achieve this or that.

Here is an example:

Martin P. comes to one of my seminars, which deals with overcoming sabotage programs. I am asking the Why question, wording it as we did here, and he answers it for himself on a piece of paper. After he finishes, he looks up, mystified, and then smiling. He shares feedback with the group, which changes his whole life: "Now it's clear to me that I want to achieve all these things because they make me a better person. They require growth and self-realization. To achieve the goal seems not to be important anymore... the goals themselves change all the time. Or, I may achieve a goal but not feel what I thought I should feel at the end because it's a goal, something outside myself. But ... the personality I develop while achieving the goals... that is what it's all about. This is what counts in the end."

The expression on his face shows surprise and enthusiasm. Two very important supercharged energies that he can, from now on, use. He has understood precisely the heart of asking the "Why" question this way: it's about what you harvest while you are walking the path, not about reaching the destination. The journey IS the destination.

Why is this so important?
Oh, look. Now I am asking the Why question!

I have a reason:
I'm inviting you to become aware of something crucial! You may have allowed fear of not achieving your goals to block you from taking a first step.

Do you see now how much there is to harvest on the way, which makes the journey worthwhile, regardless of whether you ultimately achieve the original goal?

Conclusion:
'W' questions are useful when you want to motivate yourself or to help you develop awareness of something within yourself.

Used this way, they can create real miracles.

- Have you satisfactorily answered the questions up to this point?

Then we can go ahead on our journey…

8
The Source Of Miracles
PASSIVE BELIEVERS VS. ACTIVE FAITH BUILDERS

Are you among the people who say, "Seeing is believing"?

What does this thought create in you? Does it give you power? Or does it create a dependency inside you? Are you waiting for some outside force that will give you something to believe in?

I think "Seeing is believing" makes you dependent.

It takes away your power, and puts you in a passive role... it makes you inert.

Something outside of you is active; you are passive.

I call the people who choose this kind of belief Passive Believers.

Consider this metaphor:

Let us think of humans as creatures who can only see a certain frequency with only a limited version of reality. This limited frequency, this limited vision, their eyes, would then determine how big or small their reality is and establish the strength of their beliefs.

- Do you like that?
- Do you believe that?

Where's your power in this situation? Isn't the seer here put into a passive role, whereas the eye is given an active task?

I believe that this takes away your power, the power to believe in things that are beyond the capability of the eye to see.

If you choose to stay in that passive role, this is just fine. It's your decision.

If you feel uncomfortable, unhappy and discouraged... Wouldn't it be more empowering to decide to take a more active part in your ability to see and believe? This is what I call an Active FaithBuilder.

Deciding to be an Active FaithBuilder would place you into a different reality where you know that your eye can only receive a certain frequency range, and you know there is a reality, an experience, beyond that limited reach.

- What if you could invite the PassiveBeliever inside you to look through the eyes of the Active FaithBuilder?
- What would you see then?

And if you can't do it right now, you might want to use a trick... choose at least two people who you know believe in you. Who have faith in you no matter what!

Ask those people:

- Why do you have faith in me?
- What is it about me, that Inspires your faith in me?

Now take their answers and try to look at yourself through their eyes.

- What do you see?
- What new faith do you actively create in that

moment?

- What would you do differently, when you look at yourself through their eyes, than you might have done before?
- What kind of new faith would you develop, seeing yourself this way?
- How would these experiences influence you in the role of being an Active FaithBuilder?
- How would that be beneficial for your future?

9

The Source Of Miracles
THE "HOW" WILL SHOW UP

I have read a quote somewhere that goes something along the lines of "When everybody makes the same mistake, then it is considered a truth."
I want to invite you to look harder:

- How often do you just repeat something that you have heard and act as if it was a fact, without ever questioning it?

John G. came to one of my workshops. He realized that he is standing in his own way. My observation was that he was stuck in some sort of problem trance, repeating the same sentences over and over again (which is a very popular habit by the way...). A part of this was that he wanted to open a practice, but he hadn't done anything about it because he didn't know how. So his story was that as long as he didn't know how to do it perfectly, he wasn't even going to start.

Ah. Isn't that interesting?

He didn't know how to do it so he didn't do anything at all.

This is a very common phenomenon. It is often prioritized in importance, very high on the Top Ten Most Cited Reasons to do nothing, right behind, "I'll believe it when I see it."

I'm presenting this somewhat tongue-in-cheek, not to make a joke of John's story, but to diffuse the energy of those sentences that we think are so powerful in our lives.

Before you allow a thought to dis-empower you, dis-empower it.

When we look at it together, we realize that the most important thing is to make a decision. The next step would be that you stick to it by going into action.

So when John chooses not to act because he doesn't know 'How', he takes the power away from his decision and from himself. Instead he could stay in his power by sticking to his decision and using that momentum as the first step towards his goal.

This action would move him forward. And from his new position, he would have a perspective he would not have had before.

I want to share my conclusion with you and inspire you to move forward with this thought "Stick to your decision and take any first step to energize your choice". The 'How' will show up once you've made this first step and are walking on the path towards your goals. Give yourself the permission to try different directions – directions that allow you to make "mistakes" and to learn from them.

Questions that might help you:

- How can you show your commitment to your decision?
- How would that impact you?
- Which first step could you take today to get a little

bit closer to your goal, independent of what comes next?
- How would you like to reward yourself for taking that very first step?

Usually the biggest step is the first one!

10

The Source Of Miracles
THE REWARD: SUBCONSCIOUS SUSTENANCE

When we have an experience that certain behaviors provide certain rewards we are willing to repeat this behavior over and over again. We repeat it in order to feel comfortable, while we try very hard to avoid situations that make us feel uncomfortable, by not even going there. This is saved in our limbic system, a part of our brain, which I will go into in more detail later in this book.

So when it appears not to be worth it, we won't do it. Or, to look at it differently we're preprogrammed beings!

Whenever we want to create a change, our brain automatically searches for experiences, or negative emotions in our past that would threaten our security and survival in taking this new cause of action.

If it finds something it would probably try to avoid in any way possible making these changes. They might be perfectly appropriate NOW but the brain will not be able to see the reward.

To ensure that behavioral changes are connected to rewards, we need to create them so your whole being will support the continuation of the new pattern.

What do you think?

If you agree, and this is your reality as well, then I invite you to think about how you would like to reward yourself for the changes you are making. It is worth it to reward your self for even small steps. For partial solutions and ActionsOnTheWay.

Planning the reward in advance is such a powerful factor that it will energize your decisions and will also count as a step in itself.

Let us work with John and his new practice as an example. Let us say that he has determined to do something for his project every day, which is a very effective decision that you can use for every goal.

Today he looked for a location for his office, and he rewarded himself in the evening by going to the cinema watching one of his favorite movies.

What would help you to reward yourself and to feel the power of your actions?

I have a suggestion for you: Create a plan of partial steps for each and every day, which are doable. Then reward yourself appropriately for this deed. You enjoy this reward and then you let it go. Now you have time for other things. The next day, take time to create the next partial step. And so on…

If you do that long enough (let's say 21 days) your brain learns that this kind of change is connected to something comfortable and embraces new experiences more and more.

- For what would you like to reward yourself today?
- What does that reward look like?
- When should the reward take place?
- What would you like to reward yourself for next?
- How?

What do you think?
- How would you benefit from letting go after completing each step in order to do something else?

11
The Six Levels Of Being Consciously Miraculous
THE MIRACLE OF THE SIX

Now that we know about the Source of Miracles, let us look again, broadening our view to the six levels of human existence.

Let us use a metaphor here to help us think about these levels, and how they interact. Life on earth takes place on six continents very similar to how we experience life: on the physical, emotional – energetic, mental, systemic (family systems; working systems; relationships) and soul levels.

On mother earth, the continents are connected and disconnected by the oceans; the level of human existence that is outside of time & space similarly connects and disconnects all the levels within us.

Everything that we experience, how we interpret it, and what these interpretations do with us, takes place in these six levels. Every disease, every healthy condition, this is the place where we find the root causes for problems and challenges, but also their solutions. These six levels are like a miracle themselves. Maybe we're not always aware of it, especially when we're not feeling well.

The miracle of the physical level:

Your body still functions somehow, even when it's off kilter. It can compensate a long time, appearing as if everything is okay, and only when it can't handle anymore, it starts showing weaknesses. When this happens, we tend to get angry because our body doesn't function, as we are accustomed.

Instead, we should be grateful that it has dealt with our neglect for such a long time.

- Would you like to do that?
- If yes, what would change for you and your body?

So this is the miracle of the physical level: Shouldn't we be grateful for the body's support, the home it provides and its vitality right up to the point where it 'Has' to show us its needs.

- What would you like to thank your body for?

The miracle of the emotional-energetic level:

For me it's that our emotions and our energy flow are connected to each other. When we are boiling with anger, all of a sudden, we have more power in order to defend ourselves. If we're feeling depressed, we have relatively low energy levels so that we can't hurt ourselves.

Isn't that wondrous?

- What does that mean for you?
- How would you like to use your emotions to impact your energy?
- What kind of emotions would they be?
- How would they influence your overall energy?

The miracle of the mental level:
Our mind is lightning fast in evaluating things. If it were not so capable, you could not survive, because you couldn't distinguish a dangerous snake from a harmless fly.

- What would happen if you consciously used your ability to discern what is good for you or what is not?
- How would that affect your day-to-day choices?

The miracle of the systemic level:
We are driven to think, to feel, and to do things in our lives that we would never do, had we been born in a different place, time, or even into a different family. At the beginning of your life, it is important to belong, in order to grow into independence, when you can step into your own truth.

Suppose you felt free to be in your own truth:

- What choices would you make in your present life?
- In what areas might you choose differently than your parents or grandparents did, but you didn't dare until now?

The miracle of the soul level:
We are spiritual individuals. Our experience of life on planet earth is enhanced by the insights and wisdom we receive when we attend the nourishment of our spirits. Some might say that people who immerse in spirituality are doing so to avoid "reality." But for me, personally, it is "spirituality avoidance" to only see the mundane, and to deny the metaphysical level of life.

- How could you benefit by opening up your view to include spiritual answers?

- When, for you, does it seem to be more sensible to look more to spirituality and when does it seem to serve to attend the material level?
- What might result if you played with the answers to the previous questions?

The miracle of the level outside of time and space:

We are capable of being intuitive and of communicating and exchanging information non-verbally. This binds us together as a group and protects us from the outside when needed. It allows the interdependence among us to shine when we react as a community or create something that exceeds the reach of the individual and extends the power of the whole.

- When have you caught yourself just Knowing, intuitively?
- What would happen if you consciously used this intuitive Knowing?
- With whom have you already experienced non-verbal communication in your life?

12

The Six Levels Of Being Consciously Miraculous
THE SIX LEVELS MIRRORED IN YOUR DECISIONS

As I mentioned before, all six levels are always active, and always work together... even in the process of handling decisions. As our decisions have such an immense influence on us, I would like to make a journey with you, through the levels, to illuminate how your decisions reflect those levels within.

I say: Other than recognizing a truly strengthening decision just in your head you realize it on all levels.

What do you think?

On the physical level, you recognize Truly Strengthening Decisions in your posture, your attitude and your view. Your posture will straighten, stabilize, and balance. Your view gets sharper, clearer, and more focused. You feel taller, and notice it when you look at others.

- How did you feel in your body after having made a powerful decision?
- What created this sensation?

On the emotional-energetic level, you recognize Truly Strengthening Decisions in an increase in energy and motivation to put things into action. You feel in the flow and your emotions provide power. This doesn't necessarily mean that the situation you are in would be described as positive… for example, an emotion can arise that brings you more in connection with yourself, thereby giving you access to inner resources that might have been hidden. This is how I experienced the loss of my father. The intensity of energy that was unleashed kicked off my willingness to move forward in my life.

- When did you experience something like this?
- What did it unleash in you?
- What do you think would have happened if you didn't go through the experience?

On the mental level you recognize a Truly Strengthening Decision in that you make a commitment – some sort of inner contract with yourself – around it. This includes the sense that you would give everything for the achievement of this purpose. All else pales in priority; no distraction will be brooked; this takes up the vanguard position in your thought processes and all thoughts and ideas that may follow must pass muster, or they're out.

- What is it that makes you want to commit completely?
- What forces that work against this would you have to eliminate so that you can wholly live this decision?
- What forces support this?

On the soul level, a Truly Strengthening Decision can be recognized by an overwhelming feeling that this is precisely the contribution you could give to the universe and be completely at peace with yourself.

- What would you have to do to give yourself the feeling of doing exactly what your soul longs for?
- What uplifts you to a higher level of your soul expression?
- What would create the greatest version of your self?

I believe you are accessing your true soul decisions when you choose a place that is big enough for your soul. Yes. You read that correctly. BIG enough! Most people make the "mistake" of choosing a place that's too small... and then the soul feels like chopped liver... and it won't care at all about stepping into that small place! Ha ha ha. I love this picture! The soul blows you a raspberry, and says, "This is absolutely beneath my dignity." And it's right.

- Which place would be big enough for your soul?
- How would your soul show you that you have chosen the right place?

On the systemic level, you can recognize a Truly Strengthening Decision in that it might give you a bad conscience but you feel good about it nevertheless. The bad conscience comes up because your decision might create distance between you and a certain group or person or reality... but at the same time, you feel well and in good conscience about yourself. You feel in integrity with yourself and the desire to manifest the new situation remains intact.

You end up feeling lighter and joyful because this kind of decision really belongs to you. It gives you the feeling of growth, and of being on the right path. The old 1972 song Garden Party by Ricky Nelson comes up: "you know you, you can't please everyone, so you've got to please yourself."

You know you will be able to handle the bad conscience parts more easily because of how distinctly this addresses your own gifts… and in the long run you harvest dignity and respect, even with others, because you don't seek to please others.

- What does this mean for you?
- What pours through you, demanding a place in your life?
- Who won't like this decision?
- What effect does that have on you?
- How would you like to see yourself react?
- What would develop from this decision in your life, in the short run?
- What would develop from this decision in your life, in the long run?

On the level beyond time and space, a Truly Strengthening Decision can be recognized in the resulting attraction of all that serves the decision. Here, a saying comes to my mind from Benjamin Franklin 'God helps those who help themselves'.

- What does this saying mean to you?

To me it means that you attract help and support because you take responsibility for yourself. You adjust your focus to receive information, which in turn helps you progress, while sending out information, which affects how other people react towards you.

For example:
You make a decision that you want to learn to sing.

You look up all the music schools in your area and filter out the one's that please you most. You feel a resonance with the style in which they present themselves.

1. You send out your intention (learn to sing).
2. You receive their intention (we do this well).
3. You work together so well, because they had been looking for someone just like you to work with!

- When have you had the experience of making a Truly Strengthening Decision and the universe has helped you to fulfill it?
- How did your life unfold after you made the decision
- How could you repeat these experiences?
- What do you think a truly weakening decision might be?
- Does this even exist?

I think yes. I think a truly weakening decision is a decision, which does not connect you with yourself and takes away your power; rather it is projected on you from the outside. It doesn't have anything to do with your free will and your ability to consciously take on responsibility for yourself.

- How do you see it?
- What percentages of your decisions are truly strengthening? Truly weakening?
- What percentage of strengthening vs. weakening would you like to see in your life?
- How can you achieve that new balance?

13

Our Bodyhouse: The Constant Place For Miracles

OUR BODY IS A PERFECT SURVIVAL EXPERT

Did you ever think about this? We change our house or apartment so many times in our lives, but still we have one home that is with us from the beginning of our lives until we leave: our BodyHouse.

As long as we are living in this BodyHouse, we experience the miracles of life, which shows how extremely important this place is.

To understand how a physical miracle can happen, we don't have to study medicine; we are in our body every day anyway. It is very familiar to us!

I can imagine that you will already know the things I will now describe to you.

For many of us, the physical level is the one with the most challenges. Why? Because the mind and the soul are often much faster than the inertial mass we live in. It's very good in its primary task, which is to avoid dying. It does this job around the clock 24/7.

The body is constantly looking out for potential danger, and alerts us when something suspicious arises: This is called...

... The fear-freeze-fight-flight-mechanism (4f-m):

First we get alarmed by something that could be threatening, FEAR arises often without being aware of it in that moment, our body FREEZES to pretend we're dead (like threatened lizards when they were spotted by the eagle), we FIGHT if necessary and when this doesn't work we try to run away (FLIGHT response) – or the other way around...

... Which is an automatic survival response, showing up in our bodies as:

- TEETH CLENCH to protect our head, mobilize power reserves and appear more threatening
- NECK HAIR RISING to avoid our head could be cut off
- TAIL (COCCYX) RETRACTION to gain more tension in our Cranial-Sacral system, which contains our brain and spinal cord protecting them against injuries
- BODY ROTATION to be optimally protected against 'strikes' and to get ready to fight or flee if necessary

All of this happens in an instant. These postures protect our nervous system, especially our head – because the body knows that when we 'lose our head' we die! This is why the system does all it can to keep our head on our shoulders at any price to it's self, which explains why so many people have recurrent issues with their Atlas, the first cervical vertebra supporting our head. (In Greek mythology, Atlas was the primordial Titan who supported the heavens.)

In my private practice, I see my clients stuck in the 4f-response constantly. They complain about clenching their teeth at night, or recurring neck problems, issues with their backs, or not being able to shut down. They have difficulties to fall or stay asleep, develop weight and digestion issues, concentration problems and always feel as if they were in a permanent state of red alert.

- In what way do you recognize reactions like this?
- What happens in your body?

In Stone Age, our body got rid of the tension and high adrenaline level (stress hormone) caused by stress: We went into appropriate actions like fighting or running away. Nowadays we still show the same stress reactions of ancient times but we don't act accordingly.

We would never fight with our dentist just because he seems to threaten us with a drill. (Even though we might have thought about it…)

Instead we keep the stress inside.

When the stress gets too much for our body, it doesn't turn off the fear-fight-flight reaction any more and stays frozen, even though the situation that caused the reaction initially may be over.

It thinks: "Who knows when this might come up again? I'd rather stay in this state, then I'm ready for anything." Often this condition exists for years or even decades. In kinesiology, we talk about the metaphor of the overflowing water barrel.

This concept is that stress drops into our bodies like rain into a water barrel, drop by drop until our body can no longer compensate. We reach the capacity point, and all of a sudden the whole thing overflows… not just the last drop, but rivers of past stress, strain, pain and hurt. Our body then goes into de-compensation and starts to show all kinds of issues and symptoms.

Of course, not all of our past experiences are equally important. Here it is necessary to prioritize in order to empty our metaphorical water barrel effectively.

- What do you think? How full is your barrel right now?
- What could you do about it, yourself?
- What would fill the barrel again?
- What would you do to make sure it doesn't fill up again?

14

Our Bodyhouse: The Constant Place For Miracles
SPRING CLEANING AS A MIRACLE

Pam comes to my practice. She feels desperate and totally stressed and can't calm down anymore. Her husband, who is also my client, has sent her to me, saying he can't take it anymore. She is somewhat skeptical and explains to me that she doesn't really believe in this type of treatment. As we find out later, she actually had no idea what type of treatment this is.

Nevertheless, she is experiencing tension in her jaw, her neck and shoulders are as hard as stone, and she has lumbago, sleeping disorders and fatigue. She is also gaining weight without understanding why, and she feels an inability to concentrate. Besides that she starts to panic about every little thing, which is unusual for her. Her husband suffers as well because her libido is reduced.

Pam has already been to the masseuse and chiropractor, and has experienced some improvement but the symptoms return.

Having so many kinds of different issues, she assumes she will need a lot of sessions to treat them.

I explain to Pam that her body is like a house with many rooms, electricity, and fuses. What has happened in her house is that the main fuse has blown… and this has an automatic impact on all the other rooms, similar to a chain reaction.

This doesn't mean that we need to go from room to room and check every single lamp in the house, or replace every bulb because this wouldn't help at all!

We have to go directly to the main fuse box, take care of the blown fuse, which would automatically restore the system.

I ask her how this sounds and she replies, "Oh. That explains a lot. I was wondering why I had so many different systems all of a sudden, because actually nothing dramatic happened. Now it makes sense."

I offer to do a body organization that works mainly on the nervous system, which is the electrical system of the BodyHouse. The same principle as replacing the main fuse applies here, all you have to know is where to go in the body to create the same effect… the change is instant and you feel it immediately.

She asks me how this differs from the chiropractic alignments she has already had. I tell her, "A chiropractor is like the builder of the house. I am more like the electrician." This explains why, even though she had good work done on her body, the problems recurred – the electrical system had not been addressed. This would also explain why the massage work was not integrated into her body completely, because the nerves connect to the muscles and provide electrical impulses. So without addressing the electrical system (nervous system) the musculature cannot work economically and uses way too much energy partially explaining her fatigue.

She says, "Oh! That sounds interesting. I can't wait to try it" as she lies on the treatment table to experience me tidying up her system.

- I connect what needs to be reconnected creating a re-alignment, and the tension disappears from her muscles
- I interrupt her frozen fear, flight, fight and stress patterns
- I straighten her spine and remove the tension from her jaw
- I align all her joints, balance her pelvis, and help her body to find its center

I explain to her that in this first session, we address the foundation and structure of the house. In the next session, we will stabilize the work we did today, then go further into the house, do a little "interior design" with acupressure-reflexology techniques and then focus on the "roof" with cranial-sacral osteopathy.

The body equivalents are:
The meridians, organs, glands, brain, head and jaw area.

What else is important?
I say to Pam: "Being stuck in this 4f-mechanism, you feel easily afraid of tiny little situations. This part of the barrel is too full as well and it doesn't take a lot to cause an overflow. Besides that your system shut down your metabolism and your sexuality. Why? You haven't got time to go to the toilet or sleep with somebody when you are about to fight or to run away. Your exhaustion and pain are partly a consequence of permanently using way too much energy to fulfill the daily physical tasks, which results in not having enough energy for your regeneration and reparation processes."

I also inform her of possible future challenges that could be avoided by reorganizing her body: "If your joints are not aligned over a long period of time you may develop osteoarthritis because of the wear and tear on your cartilages."

What is the body organization?

The Willow Treatment System Body Organization is based on Dr. Carl Ferreri's Neural Organization Technique, or NOT for short. I have had to change and refine some of its protocols for the needs of my clients over the years. People are always happily astonished at the speed it works, reporting feeling lighter, centered, grounded and effortlessly more upright in general.

Pam, who was skeptical at the beginning, is now absolutely happy and eager to continue, but I suggest that she gives her body time to integrate what we have done so far, returning in ten days so we can check what has happened in the interim.

Ten days later she returns as I suggested and I ask her how she's feeling. She says she was initially feeling pain free, but after about a week, some of the pain returned but not anywhere near its original intensity.

Based upon her feedback, and confirmed with kinesiological muscle tests, we discover we must dig deeper into her past to find old forgotten traumas she was still carrying around and were saved in her body.

For example:
- A sporting accident when she was young
- An inordinate number of dental treatments
- A birth trauma: Born with the umbilical cord wrapped around her neck

After another body organization in our second session, she feels relief for months. She returns when she feels a buildup of stress again, but happy to report that she has lost 10 pounds and regained her focus.

She asks me to explain once more and I do by telling her that when her body is not frozen in the fear-fight-flight-mechanism any more, it doesn't have to slow down its metabolism and build up 'fat reserves for hard times' and normal metabolism can resume.

Her concentration has improved because of the cranial and jaw work balancing the skull and allowing the brain to relax, improving both brain function and blood circulation.

And her husband is happy because her libido improved as well.

In the meantime she comes twice a year for checkup and realignment, which I call 'a spring cleaning for the BodyHouse'.

Now back to you, dear reader:
- Do you see yourself in Pam's story?
- How would you notice that your barrel is overflowing?
- What kind of spring cleaning or tidying up do you think you need?

When our body is capable of switching from the active modus in the autonomous nervous system (sympathetic) during the day into the regeneration and digestion modus (parasympathetic) in the night it provides the necessary conditions for self-reparation and for 'recharging our batteries'.

Our bodies can only heal in the parasympathetic modus. This is why we need more sleep when we get a cold, for example.

There is something else: Scientists (Dr. Garjajev and Team) found out that our DNA reacts to relaxation where it performs one of its many tasks that of creating spontaneous self-healing.

If you want to participate in your own healing process, my tip for you would be to make sure you get enough 'regeneration time'!

- How can you use this for yourself, your health and your healing processes?

15
E-MOTION-ERGY
EVERYTHING IS ENERGY

WE ARE ENERGY! And so is everything we deal with, like our cells, emotions, diseases, health, thoughts, relationships…

I think you get the idea…!

The energy in our human body manifests in three expressions.

- The aura, or morphogenetic field
- Meridians, or acupuncture pathways
- Chakras, or energy centers

All three energetic areas are connected and influence each other accordingly.

The aura is our overall energy field. It penetrates our body cells and extends beyond our physical boundaries. As with the meridians and chakras, information is saved here. Some people believe this information can come from this or other lives. The aura is a vibration field and acts like a protective shield. It can be very, very big or very, very small, depending on our life force and spiritual consciousness.

- If we're unwell, it may collapse.
- If we're healthy or enlightened, it is well developed and impenetrable.
- If there are fissures, holes, or it has imbalances we can experience problems, such as illnesses, mental confusion, emotional breakdowns, and challenges in our soul.

When we are in a relationship with someone else, energetic connections are built between our aura and the morphogenetic field of the other person. In addition, we are connected to the collective and universal energy field.

- What could you do to improve your energy field?
- What benefits are there from doing so?
- What could you do to spruce up the energetic interaction between you and others?

Now let's look at the meridians together. They are energy-rivers flowing through our bodies, carrying well-documented acupuncture points.

We have fourteen main meridians. Sometimes they can be too empty, full, or blocked, resulting in not feeling well or even full-scale sickness.

Tip: If you want to treat yourself well, you can tap certain acupuncture points on a regular basis. Look for books on the Emotional Freedom Technique (EFT).

So. Generally speaking, we can say that our energetic system always reacts first when something is out of balance before being manifested on a physical level.

- How do you discern when something is not right on the energetic level?

My personal opinion is that every one of us should have access to this knowledge. I give workshops in which you can learn quickly and easily to discern these things using kinesiology.

You can also discern energetic imbalances by using pulse diagnostics, aura diagnostics, etc.

This is important: If you've been through an illness or a stressful situation and things seem to be okay on the physical level please have yourself checked out on the energetic, metaphysical level to ensure full recovery.

- How can you use this information?
- Which advantages are there:
  o For you?
  o For your life?
  o For your environment?

The chakras (from Sanskrit: wheels) are energy centers in our body. While the traditional teachings describe that they are located along the spine and in the area of the head, I've found new theories about their location in the Dr. Roy Martina's book "Aquarius Chakras".

This motivated me to do my own research. Here are my hypotheses: I found similar chakras to those Dr. Martina talked about, and I realized something else… a difference in the energy flows of men and women. The energy flow of men is like a halo whereas the energy flow of women is like a water wheel.

A full description of these systems is beyond the scope of this book, but you can already find some information about it in my publications about Chakracise (Active Yoga Meditation), as well as in Chakracise events. A book about this subject will follow in the future.

- How can you influence your energy centers in a positive way?

You can cleanse, energize, and harmonize your chakras by meditation. Also effective are breathing techniques, moving your body, listening to relaxing music, aromatherapy, reading uplifting literature… and much more.

- How can that help you?

It can help you solve issues of the past, and invite you to manifest new and more useful behavioral and emotional patterns into your physical and energetic system and your life in general.

It can help you learn life lessons effortlessly and not get stuck in outdated programs that affect you without you being aware of them.

- What kind of outdated programs do you need to get rid of?
- Which meditation, relaxation, or breathing techniques could help you?
- What would be the first sign that you have taken out some of the trash?

16
E-MOTION-ERGY
GO AS DEEP AS IT TAKES

We are in the middle of the Willow Treatment System Practitioner Training.

The task is to learn how to tailor a treatment on a metaphysical level.

Two students, Glen and Kim, pair up to practice together. They want to find out where Kim's energy system is blocked, which could eventually make it hard for her to talk to people.

Kim wants to be able to treat clients and finally wishes to dispel this communication block for good.

They are using Systemic Dialoguing, a communication technique that I developed from parts of the systemic constructivism technique by various therapists in Germany and Italy, like Prof. Dr. Fritz B. Simon amongst others and solution-focused brief therapy, developed by Steve de Shazer and Insoo Kim Berg.

This technique is designed to allow them to get access to Kim's hidden resources and probable root causes to construct possible optimal solutions to her communication issues.

With the help of kinesiology muscle testing techniques that will involve the integration of the subconscious into the process and by using specially produced Willow System manuals they can operate on a broader spectrum of information, beyond that of the conscious level and verify if their proposed explanations to Kim's timidity are right or wrong.

They find blockages in the throat chakra, the aura and in the kidney meridian. In Kim's case, the throat chakra explains the communication problem. In the aura they find a disturbance in the I/You relationship, and in the kidney meridian they find evidence of fears about communicating with others.

As they go deeper, they discover that a trauma in Kim's past is connected to her blockages. In the past, she was strongly punished for presenting her opinion. Her metaphysical system has then saved this negative information and installed an additional warning light for the future so that Kim will react in time to protect her life if she should ever get in a situation like that again.

What is being described here is very common.

It doesn't matter if we have experienced the trauma in this, or in other lives if you believe in reincarnation. Our system wants to protect us from negative experiences, but also, very often, it thereby restricts us from living the positive ones. Only information that fits into this traumatized consciousness gets through. All the good energy that we need for vitality doesn't reach us either and seems to be inaccessible. We feel isolated, alone, and disconnected.

- How could you regain your access to the good energy life is offering you?

Intention, meditation and willpower are the keys to

attracting good energy and through metaphysical filtering; you can leave everything that's negative outside of your system.

- What else could you do?

Suppose you were in Kim's situation. In her mind she has the sensation of fear in relationship to her environment, which makes her words stick in her throat. No matter if the situation is a real threat, or not, her system perceives it as threatening warning her to secure her survival, because that's what it's designed for. This warning may have served her in the past, but now it's become a blockage.

- In what way do you see yourself in Kim's story?
- How could you take care of finding these blockages and resolving them?
- What do you think you might do differently if they were already cleared?

In Kim's case, it was necessary to dig deep enough to find the trigger for her blockages.

This is not always the case.

Sometimes our systems are so ready for solutions that no contribution is made by digging up the bones of the past. That's why it's important to go as deep as it takes to create a positive change, and stop at the right time to ensure that what we have found can show its effects.

My students learn to distinguish this principle in every treatment case by case.

Kim needed to know where her problems were and why they were there. After that, all Glen needed to do was to test out the optimal combination of solutions which included EFT meridian-tapping techniques, breathing exercises, and chakra cleansing to help release her blockages.

- How would you notice that you have to go deeper in your own solution process in order to effect real change?
- How would you do that?

I don't want to hear: "I don't know enough to answer this question!"

Dive deep down into the depths of your soul for the answers that are there, give yourself time to find them and the space they need.

- How would you notice that it's time to go into action and stop deep sea diving?

My answer is this: It's time to stop, when any additional information strips power from you, rather than adding to it.

- Do you sometimes catch yourself digging deeper in order NOT to go into action?
- Do you catch yourself sometimes digging deeper as a form of procrastination?

Ah! Interesting …

17
E-MOTION-ERGY
RIDING THE LIGHT-WAVES

As I mentioned before our DNA sends and receives information what the scientists call hyper-communication. In order to do this the DNA uses light-waves. This was intensively researched by the German bio-physicist Prof. Fritz Albert Popp.

- Where does the light go when it leaves our body?

DNA messages navigate through our morphogenetic field and that of the universe. If our aura is clear and healthy, our chakras are cleansed and our meridians balanced, we send and receive clear messages. It is more likely to interpret information correctly and use it accordingly.

Another powerful effect of being a light transmitter & receiver is that it also means that we can look at our emotional and energetic states as information, processing them to maintain clarity. We radiate light that is acknowledged and mirrored back a thousand fold.

In Kriya Yoga, an ancient technique that accomplishes

oneness between breath and soul, the chakras are compared to the petals of the lotus flower. When we take this picture and use it for us as human beings, it can tell us much about how we can use any kind of so-called 'negative' emotion for our highest good, and by doing that, have a positive influence on our DNA.

As an example, suppose you were worried about money.

As you know, worrying is just energy. So handle it as energy, no more, no less.

Worrying can be compared to mud that the lotus flower is rooted in, it's very heavy and definitely not clear. Just as the lotus flower grows in its full beauty from this mud, you can use your emotional mud as super fertilizer to grow. No matter how you are feeling, you can always treat this emotional sludge as a resource that nourishes you instead of being buried by it.

This gives you a totally different kind of freedom to deal with any emotion.

So, you were worried about money...

- How would you like to deal with it?

This would be my tip: Remember that you are like the lotus, pulling the nutrients from the mud to create beauty. The lotus would never allow the mud to pull it down, and neither will you. Instead use the energy of the mud to pull yourself up and show your colors above the surface.

To be able to do that, why not accept feeling worried. When you fight it, it fights back. When you deny it, it shows its power over you. This has got nothing to do with fatalism it's generating a place of inner freedom from where you can make totally new decisions.

These decisions will come from a 'place of power' instead of a 'place of fears'.

They create a 'constructive energy field' instead of a 'destructive battlefield'.

This has an impact on the vibration and frequency of your own morphogenetic field and your DNA response. Your molecules receive and send out a message of 'hope' and 'resources', which shifts your focus of attention from 'problem' to 'solution'.

It shifts your body from being 'frozen' to being 'in motion'.

Instead of feeling heavy, you are riding the light wave.

Looking again at yourself and the way you deal with worry, or any other so-called negative emotions:

- How would you deal with them now?
- What kind of different results would you get now?
- How can you remind yourself to ride the light wave in your every day life?

18
A Mentastic World
ACTIVATING
MIRACULOUS INTELLIGENCE

First of all, I take my hat off to our intelligence, which is very active in all of us. Look at what it's doing all the time! It learns, evaluates and assesses life dangers to support our survival, makes logical conclusions and constructs plans for the future. It is creative and imaginative. It makes and rejects decisions by the minute.

- What would happen if we used this genius inside us to work FOR us instead of against us?

Why am I asking this question? I have observed, the more intelligent and talented someone is, the more potential they have, the more they are in danger of using this quantity of qualitative intelligence against themselves.

Our inherent creativity is often guided down paths that unleash the 4f-mechanism rather than encouraging our own productivity.

Do you remember?
The power that creates is the power that destroys.

- How would you notice that you are using your intelligence against yourself?
- How would you turn it around and use it FOR you?

What do you need to create Miraculous Intelligence?

To create Miraculous Intelligence, it is necessary to see that what you think and how you judge someone or something may not be right. An intelligent "I don't know if my judgment is really correct," and taking a new look with another sense of value and a different perspective will set off unbelievably precious insights.

- Which of your judgments are serving you?
- Which are harming you?
- How could you transform the harmful judgments to ones that serve you?
- And then what would change?

I hear regularly from clients and seminar participants that they would prefer to not judge at all.

But how can our intelligence not make judgments?
It's like forbidding the train driver to drive the train…

My opinion is that to create Miraculous Intelligence you need to accept the judgments you make, but choose to deal with them in a different way.

Two things are necessary to accomplish this:

1. To acknowledge that our intelligence is limited.
2. To interpret its interference as simply a comment, not the absolute fixed truth.

Something like, "Ah! That's what you think, dear mind. That's interesting! What else is new?"

Put yourself in a position where you can spread inviting curiosity in which your intelligence is given a good place, but not given power over you. Allow it to be part of the team like the heart, emotions and soul, but don't unduly venerate it.

- What do you think about that?
- What does your intelligence think?
- What does your heart think?
- What does your soul think?
- Is there anyone else that has something to say?
- What changes if you use your intelligence this way?

Are you aware of why your intelligence acts the way it does?

Actually, in its heart of hearts, it's afraid. It's absolutely terrified of being kicked off the team. It's frightened that somebody, somewhere, will find out that it doesn't know as much as it pretends to know and that it has trouble keeping up with the rest of the team.

It thinks:
Attack Is The Best Form Of Defense!

Our intelligence accepts something only as true that which it understands in its limited boneheaded world.

So, now that we know that our intelligence is afraid of losing its place, we can calm it down by telling it, "You will always be part of the team. You don't have to be perfect to please us… we will never throw you out. You don't have to know all the time; you don't have to understand all the time. We can help. We always listen to you and we might not always agree, but that doesn't mean you have to fear anything. We work together as a team, and you are part of that team."

- When will you be ready to open yourself up for things that are beyond your intelligence?
- How would you benefit?
- How would you show your intelligence that it would always be a valued part of the team?

19
A Mentastic World
THE POWER OF CONVICTION

Convictions have a very strong influence on us because they become emotionally loaded. We believe in them even when this is not understandable for other people. We can use this intense power in the areas of our lives where we suffer from a lack of conviction.

For example:
You might want to have the conviction that you are able to achieve your goals.

- What do you think you would have to do to convince yourself a 'little bit more' that you can achieve your goals, somehow?

The word 'somehow' is purposely chosen here. Many people believe that they can either achieve their goals in certain ways, or not at all.
The times of this very popular 'either-or'-thinking are over! Now the time has come to live 'as-well-as' solutions.

The word 'somehow' gives you more flexibility, because when Plan A doesn't work, there can be a Plan B, Plan C etc.

So, instead of giving up your goal, you give up the belief that there is only one 'How'.

- What is the first indication that you are becoming comfortably convinced that you can achieve your goal?
- What other indications are there?
- And what else?
- How does this 'little bit more' conviction inside you motivate you to continue?
- What becomes possible now, that wasn't possible before?

20

A Mentastic World
THE MIND: "A GLIMMER THAT GIVES THE BODY A SOUL"

When we want to fulfill mental miracles then it's absolutely necessary to set your mind to the glimmer that gives the body a soul. This glimmer gives your thinking a sense, or a non-sense; it builds opinions and convictions, and creates memories to remember. It helps to build up our consciousness and awareness, while supporting us in our decision-making processes.

Our mind has three levels:

1. The subconscious
2. The conscious
3. The super conscious

The mind, the glimmer, also has physical counterparts within the brain. When information passes through our thalamus, the gateway to consciousness, it enters the neocortex, but the majority does not go through and stays in the subconscious. In this context super consciousness means that we have access to information and knowledge that goes beyond the realms of our personal consciousness and subconscious.

Our brain is divided into four parts:

1. The Neocortex – intellect and thinking
2. The Limbic System – emotions and survival (4f-mechanism)
3. The Brain Stem – basic vital life functions
4. The Cerebellum – coordination and balance

The subconscious mind influences our emotions, thinking, and actions, and thereby, our future decisions. Here, the limbic system also plays an important role, as the physical center for our feelings, affections, and survival.

In its almond-shaped Amygdala, the limbic system, as early as in the womb, can perceive so-called 'negative' emotions, like fear.

The neocortex is the part of the brain that houses the conscious mind, and develops later than the limbic system.

This is why in our formative years; let's say in the first year of our lives, we experience something negative. It would then be saved in our limbic system, because our conscious mind, the neocortex, is not yet fully developed. This negative memory can surface and be triggered by another situation later in our adult life. Suddenly we feel down, depressed, or very uncomfortable without any rational explanation for feeling that way.

What's happening here is that our neocortex wasn't able to give this emotion a home address, something like the 'save as' command on a computer, when the negative feeling originally occurred because at that time it wasn't capable of doing so. The consequence is that we feel 'something', but haven't got any rational explanation that would explain it.

Here is an example:

Mr. Jones is 46 years old when he comes to me for a session. He has anxiety, which has been tremendously improved by psychotherapy, but still there is 'something' that he can't put his finger on: He experiences panic in the dark.

We do some kinesiology muscle testing and discover that he had a brother that was two years older than him, who died in the night when he was two months old. His brother died in the same room where he was sleeping. He tells me that he has been addressing this in psychotherapy.

- So what can be done to help him move on?

We find out two things:

He didn't see any connection between his panic in the dark and the death of his brother. Now he understands. Every time it gets dark, this memory comes up from his limbic system, but doesn't have a rational home address in his conscious mind, the neocortex.

Now he can give that 'something' an address, which helps him tremendously, because his brain can assess the situation differently and he can relax. The threatening aspect vanishes and his nervous system can stop warning him at dusk, because his brother won't die again.

The second thing that we had to integrate into his treatment was a body organization, that was tailored to this dynamic, to ensure that his body didn't fall back into the 4f-mechanism in the dark. This organization helped him to align his body in the present and to put the past experience in the past where it belonged. In the meantime he feels well and holds only a loving memory of his older brother.

- What's going on inside you while you read this?
- What do you become conscious of?
- In which areas of your daily life do you experience recurring negative emotions, or even panic, which

you couldn't explain until now?
- How would you explain it now with your newfound knowledge?
- How will you deal with it from now on?

21

A Mentastic World
LACK MENTALITY
... IT'S ALL THE RAGE!

Besides Dior and Gucci, negative and limiting belief systems also belong to one of the most popular fashions of our time.

This is the time of... Lack Mentality!

Here are some examples:

- It's lonely at the top.
- No good deed goes unpunished.
- High flyers fall further.
- You can't always get what you want.
- He who hesitates is lost.
- Nothing is certain but death and taxes
- The best laid plans of mice and men...

What negative expressions do you use to shoot yourself in the foot?

By taking on collective and common values of any group, you can limit your consciousness, and by that, your whole life, without even noticing it. In the chapter on Group Consciousness I will go into this in more detail. So when your own needs and desires don't match the concept of the group your whole organism can suffer, bringing sickness and spiritual or mental problems.

Why? From a very early age our limbic system knows, that if we don't belong to the family, or any other type of group, our survival would be threatened. This is why we have such a drive to belong or to fit in. To be part of something or to be an outcast has a great power over us.

This can even go as far as disconnecting ourselves from our true needs and desires for the sake of belonging to something.

Being a breeding ground for manipulation this instinct in us to want to belong is abused every day of our lives by mass media, in our education and health system, our relationships.

In my workshop 'Step-by-Step 2U' I train people to be aware of this dynamic, and in this book, I want you to be aware of it as well. When you train your mind to be conscious of what your space is and realize when 'someone' steps over these boundaries, you can make the decision to cast this 'someone' out, filling out your space yourself to its full extent.

Let's say you're 50 years old, feeling fit and healthy. You sit down to watch TV. In the commercials you see which illnesses your age group are susceptible to. The man tells you, you should get checked out by the doctor, because there's a very good chance you may already have them all!

It's presented as if they are caring, but the intention is: 'Buy this stuff'!

- "It's in your best interest."
- "It's for your own security."
- "Stay alert …cancer, aging, danger!"

So, if you were feeling good until then you might start to think that you should get yourself check out to see if you've 'got the signs' that will show you "there's something wrong with me". This process takes away energy and directs your focus of attention on lack.

You might ask yourself: "Why do I feel so bad? I was in such a good mood before?"

Stay aware that this is not your reality and don't participate in this lack mentality and you will stay in your power. When you chose to get a check up because you want to know how good your health is, it's then your own decision. It's not being pressed on you to help the pharmaceutical industry increase their revenue, and it will have a completely different intention.

The challenge is to stay aware of what choices are yours and where you react to somebody else's choice and unnaturally make it yours. Keep observing yourself closely to find out, while you stay in the meta-level that I described earlier in the book.

My opinion is that this is the best self-protection from involuntary manipulation.

Let's take another look at this 'Lack Mentality Fashion' and its driving force, designed to make you participate. As we already know our limbic system always checks to see if our survival is threatened, it also checks whether we are an outcast, or not. If you your mindset is not conform, or synchronized with the group you are living in, you are in danger to doubt your own convictions.

- Maybe I'm wrong?
- Maybe I'm not being realistic?
- And so on…

Your system suggests, "Your survival is in danger because you are disconnecting from the group. You are now easy prey for the enemy, or wild animal attacks." The difference is that we no longer live this way. It's important to update our systems to the reality of the present day.

For instance:
"I'm different and I've a right to feel good about myself!"

- How do you feel reading this?
- How does it influence you?
- When or where did you suppress your needs and desires because they were uncomfortable to others?
- How would you like to deal with them now?
- What mindset could you choose instead of a Lack Mentality?
- What do you fear most would happen, if you made this decision?
- Which of these fears could really happen, if any?
- And then what?

We are mainly afraid of what in our 'fantasy' could happen which probably never will.

22

A Mentastic World
BE SMART
WHEN YOU'RE INTELLIGENT!

I'm assuming that you are, otherwise you would have already put away this book. Ha ha ha!

It's easy to persuade an intelligent person with a logical argument: "You need this or that because otherwise you … blah blah blah".

This is what happens to intelligent people

Your mind gets busy with so called realities that are outside of your own environment. You understand you need a certain 'THING', because they explain it well to you and it sounds logical. All of a sudden, you understand why you can't live without 'IT'. Even though there was no need for 'IT' before, they have created this need in your head. They are tricking you into devaluing your own self-sustaining power to decide, while putting your sense of judgment in question. They encourage you to giving up your power of decision on a subliminal level.

Being intelligent, the more logic that comes with a product, any kind of product and the more plausible they sound, or appear and depending on how well they are presented, the more you accept them without questioning.

Here is an example: You learn that 'studies show' that blah blah blah, and this is why you have to do blah blah blah to ensure that your survival is secured. Because of this and that reason, everybody needs this and that for their own good, not to be afraid anymore of… and for their own best welfare and safety.

At this point, I want to make it clear that I'm not against prevention or protection… but what bothers me is the way that 'THINGS' are presented and sold, using fear and a fictitious need, or lack, because of the power these emotions have over us.

- How do you feel about this?
- What is your opinion?

My favorite questions are:

- Who financed these studies that have been published, so logically?
- What happens in the brains of the intelligent people they influence?

This is what happens

1. First, you create a need.
2. Then you present something that fills it.

The theory behind this is:

- You are not enough.

For instance:

- Your body cannot do enough.
- Your effort is not sufficient.
- You don't have enough money.
- You don't have enough energy.
- Simply… blah blah blah.

So what happens is that we get disconnected from our inherent ability to perceive ourselves as fulfilled beings, so that we are constantly living in the illusion that we need something more. This makes us controllable and easily manipulated because the focus of our attention is on what we need, or seem to need… it's on lack, and not what we already 'Are':

- Complete…

Being that this is a lack that is artificially produced we can't ever really attain complete fulfillment of this illusion. Our thoughts constantly swirl around what we don't have, or haven't enough of… We then become more and more receptive to further manipulation always looking for the next thing that will make us happy, fulfilled, complete, etc.

Once an idea of Lack is out there, everybody just repeats it, without checking or testing its credibility. All of a sudden it's reality. This is how a big group of intelligent people can be controlled in a very powerful way.

The recipe is simple:

1. Take one part desire. E.g. Good health.
2. Add endless messages of impossibility of its achievement. Unless, without, only, if…
3. Pour in declarations and diagnoses. Worry, risk, and doubt…

4. Keep the mind busy. Wrapping it around the fingers of those sending out the messages…
5. Maintain a lack mentality. Until everybody is soft and malleable

- Which kind of Lack Mentality do you suffer from?
- How do you feel when you don't have these 'needs' met?
- Where do these feelings come from?
- And now, what should happen and what will you think about this new situation?
- How have you reclaimed your completeness?

So, be smart when you're intelligent and train yourself in becoming more and more mindful about what's happening around you and inside you. It's absolutely essential to live in an awareness of being your own 'source of resources' and to realize when you disconnect from this awareness by self-observation. I invite you to go even further and step into a 'knowing' that you are an endless source of resources – like you did when you were a child.

- What is the very first sign that you are about to step into lack thinking?
- How would your life change if you lived your life out of the 'knowing' that you are the resource?
- If you caught yourself falling back into lack – what would you like to do differently now?
- How do you notice that you are about to fall back into lack?
- How would you notice that you have chosen a powerful way out of it?
- What would be important in the future in order to 'know you're your greatest resource'?
- How would that new memory change your future?

Intelligent people:

- Be aware
- Be honest with yourself
- Be true to yourself

By the way, if you are one of those who always do the opposite of what others do, you are still trapped in the same dynamic, because you make your decisions based on the same reality. To be opposite doesn't mean to be free.

- Who, or what would be influenced if you were to be free?

23
A Mentastic World
THE POWER OF INTENTION

Dr. Garjajev and his team found out that the part of our gen molecule that was formerly known as 'silent' DNA (90%), is not silent at all. It contains the blueprint of communication. The DNA is capable of sending out and receiving information by creating tiny wormholes and passes it on to our conscious mind.

This would explain how intuition works.

The DNA reacts to words and intention, explaining why methods like hypnosis and affirmation have such an effect on us. Knowing this please be aware of the intention behind your mindset, what you think and say, because this can be creative or destructive.

Here's an example: Five years ago Mary came into my practice, diagnosed with cancer and the doctors were saying it didn't look good. As you can understand she was desperate and had lost all faith in herself.

We found out that she and her doctors considered that if she died it would be some kind of 'failure', making the intention behind the treatment 'to prevent dying' instead of 'creating a space for healing'.

She realized that there were lots of things she hadn't done, thinking she had all the time in the world, taking on her company's, mother's, doctor's priority, in fact everybody's priority, but her own in the way she lived her life…

What do you fear most about death?

"It might sound strange but I am afraid of dying before having experienced being ALIVE. I am scared of losing everybody and everything. This is how I lived my whole life. I never dared to fully step into my possibilities because I was always afraid of loss."

Would death be the biggest loss?

"Yes. I wasn't aware until now what a loss it would be and somehow thought I wouldn't lose so much if I didn't put so much energy into my life! The more abundant my life became the bigger the loss was going to be in death."

What's going on inside you?

"My friends have been putting pressure on me, saying that I should start to use my intention to fight death, in order to survive. Now, I feel guilty because I realize that I can't, but if I don't, I'll die. I feel trapped in a vicious circle that takes away all my power I need for healing."

What would you need to break free?

"I'd need to get away from all the pressure."

My reaction was to try something new:
"We both know that people don't want to die? What if

we looked at using your intention differently, in a way that might seem paradox? Let's see how you feel if you used your intention to embrace death as a natural consequence of being alive and then enjoy life even more. So, you don't choose to put your intention AGAINST death, but FOR life. Like you were doing martial arts where the defender uses the attacker's energy to guide the force into a direction that's not hurting him or her. How does that sound?"

She thought it made totally sense, that it was making her feel calmer and asked me to explain how the power of intention worked, as she was not really clear.

I suggested an experiment. I would massage the back of her neck three times, each time for just a minute, with a different intention for every massage without telling her my intention. Then she would give me a feedback on how she felt at the end.

1. My first intention was "Nothing will help you anyway."
2. My second was "I'm not interested in you."
3. My third was "My hands are channels providing the energy you need."

She said that in the first two massages she felt very uncomfortable and was thinking about leaving, but the third time she felt safe, comforted and happy.

By the way: She's still alive!

How would you use your intention:

- On the physical level?
- On the emotional- energetic level?
- On the mental level?
- On the group or family level?
- On the soul level?

How would you put it into action:

- Now?
- In one year?
- In five years?

Now my intention is to invite you to explore being "made in… me".

24

A Mentastic World
MADE IN... ME

Let's do a little summing up!

If you don't make up your mind, somebody else will do it for you. There are plenty of people with lots of little stickers, just dying to stick it to you:

- "Made in Hong Kong",
- "Made in Taiwan",
- "Made in America"
- Etc.

- How do we avoid this?
- How do we begin?

You make up your mind to make up your mind.

Walk with me through all the levels again:

- As you are intelligent, use your mind consciously.
- Harness the power of "I think therefore I am."

- Invite yourself to use your mind in totally new ways, let's say as a vibrant center of Creativity.
- When fuses are in, that light bulb over your head burns brighter.
- When you are in touch with your true emotions and the energy flows, it will give you access to creative thinking.

You can choose to align your thoughts with that which serves your highest purpose, with that which is fundamentally motivating.

Then, the sticker is as it should be...
- "Made In... Me."

25
Unraveling Entanglements
THE TRUTH HEALS IN THE DEPTHS

Talia comes for a private session. She explains that she's had a problem for a long time with diarrhea and weight loss, and that now, it's gotten to the point where her day to day choices are dictated by her symptoms, as she can't be too far away from a bathroom at any one time. In addition, her fear of diarrhea makes it even worse.

Nothing has helped so far!

- Do you recognize any elements of this story in your own life?
- How do you explain it, when nothing helps?

Using Systemic Dialoguing, we discover that Talia suffers from a conflict, unresolved issues with her mother and sister. Muscle testing shows us the absolute priority for her session:

- Dealing with the mother issue.

Talia tells me that for as long as she can remember, her mother has only thought of herself and has shown no interest in her. She starts to cry and then realizes that she is not crying out of sadness, but out of anger. This anger smoldering in her gut is the main cause of her diarrhea.

I invite Talia to do a little family constellation work, which was originally developed by the German psychotherapist Bert Hellinger. In the Willow Treatment System I use the fundamental ideas he presented but work with them in a totally new way.

This work deals with the weakening dynamics that exist on the subconscious level within the family or ancestry. Every member of a system present and past adds to a group's energy field, like an energetic history book, that is called the 'knowing field'.

Each system looks for compensation, affecting those who belong to the system. If at some point something disturbing happens in the past, lets say injustice, loss, or guilt the members of the system unconsciously react to it. This injustice, loss, or guilt can resurface in the present depending with whom the person is connected, entangled, or bonded with and the place he or she occupies in the family order.

In a session our task is to find weakening or sickening dynamics, turning them into strengths and resources.

In this process, I encourage my clients to give the appropriate family members a place in the room, in relationship to themselves. I check this constellation for accuracy and we look together, how person, or persons brought to the room relate to the client by there position, proximity, distance, if their standing, sitting, where they're facing, etc. From this we derive useful information that we would not get without this work. Joy and sorrow, guilt and innocence, justice and injustice can be identified and treated accordingly, so that a "good order" is created in the system, each filled with ease.

I ask Talia to bring her mother in and choose a place in

the room for her, and one for herself that feels right. We can feel the tension between Talia and her Mother immediately. Talia experiences a physical sensation – the now very familiar clenching of her stomach. This allows her to identify that the root cause of the physical symptom is the dynamic between herself and her mother.

Now I ask Talia how her mother feels. In this setting, now having this new understanding of herself Talia is able to report that her mother feels unheard, misunderstood and that no one takes her seriously.

Talia has never seen this before.

- She is quite surprised at how clear the family dynamic now seems to her, and how it is so quickly achieved!
- She sees the tangle of emotional energies that has been affecting her family's interactions for years.

This physical awareness develops out of the 'knowing field'.

So how does the session go on?

We continue with this systemic process. I invite Talia now to speak to her mother, to communicate some of how she is feeling, to speak out her inner truth and express to her mother what she would have told her already, if there had been space for the words before. She does so and realizes that she already feels better. In this process, she develops more understanding about herself and that of the relationship with her mother that creates more compassion, within her.

As a result, Talia develops compassion for her self and feels that her suffering is taken seriously. It is as if the adult Talia has taken the child Talia by the hand to take care of it. The adult consciousness understands now what's creating the tension in her gut and tells the child: "It has nothing to do with you, little one you are innocent you've done nothing wrong..." and the little one can relax and exhale.

Now that Talia has found this peace inside her, she develops compassion toward her mother's pain. She says to me, gently, "You know, Rita, my mother did not have an easy life. She lost her own mother when she was only seven, and was raised by a stepmother who didn't treat her very well."

So now, we can go one step further and decide to create a healing space for her mother.

This time, we bring in her grandmother, and set her in the room with Talia's mother. Now, together, we find that Talia's mother can finally break down and cry, having the benefit of the undivided attention of her own mother, who she has been missing all her life.

She finally experiences catharsis.

"Everyone is feeling happy now," says Talia and I explain to her that she has subconsciously felt the lack in her mother and has wanted to fill it. She could never give her mother what she needed from her own mother because she was just a child.

In addition, Talia realizes an improvement in her body. Her belly is now relaxed and comfortable. As she returns ten days later for another session, her symptoms have decreased by approximately eighty per cent.

She tells me that she's enjoying the relationship with her mother, whose behavior has changed automatically, because we changed the dynamic in the 'knowing field'!

We do a body organization:

In only two sessions we stabilize her new condition and all her physical symptoms disappear.

- How does this story affect you?
- What parallels can you see in your life?
- What do you wish for in your relationships to family members?
- How can you achieve it?

26
Unraveling Entanglements
YOU ARE ALSO A PRODUCT OF YOUR ENVIRONMENT

We are all a part of a system, in the beginning we are a part of the family system and later, we become parts of many other systems. Relationships with others play a very key role throughout our lives.

Bert Hellinger says that all relationships are guided by:

- Systemic order
- Bonding
- A balance between giving and receiving

In sharing these ideas, my intention is simple and clear: to invite you to explore your own thoughts and feelings while you read this.

Do you remember at the beginning of the book, I said it would be written from your point of view?

So, we won't go into too much detail here, because it's such a broad subject and there is so much literature available, if you wish to explore this area more precisely.

Systemic Order
Every system has within it a natural order that gives it strength. Consider your workplace as an example. Your team has worked well together for the last ten years. Someone new comes along and begins to act as if they were also on the job for ten years, without knowing the least bit about what the job entails. As you can imagine this would create a disturbance in the system as a whole.

This is why it is so important that we acknowledge the power of 'the rules of succession' within any system.

In a family system, 'the rules of succession' are:
The parents were there before the children existed. The exception is the patchwork family where the first marriage and the children of that family were there before the new family was founded.

In the sibling configuration the first-born is acknowledged being the first, then the second, and so on, including those infants who were stillborn or died, abortions are not included.

This birth order is important to how strong the family is as a whole. When everybody sits on their rightful chair (even though they might not always like it), the family members can feel at ease.

Sometimes, parents and children have reversed roles. This imbalance in 'the rules of succession' always has a consequence.

For example:
The child in question may feel angry, disgusted or even contempt toward the parents, feeling that their parents are weak. A further outcome could be that the child develops self-sabotage programs to punish themselves for placing themselves before the parents... this is the system trying to right itself.

In the preceding chapter, Talia's subconscious role reversal was a classic example of the previously described disturbance in 'the rules of succession'. She developed a physical symptom expressing the conflict she carried inside herself for taking on the role of a parent.

- Where can you see disturbances in 'the rules of succession' within the systems you live in?
- How do those disturbances impact your life?
- How would things change if you reclaimed your rightful place, returning the others to their appropriate positions?

Now let us look at the idea of bonding. The fact that you are born into a system automatically creates a bond between you and this system – especially between you and your mother and father. Even if you were to grow up in a different family, this bonding would have an effect on you, as it is the first you form and affects all that follow.

Within this bond is our primary avenue for the flow of love. The strength of this bond cannot be understated. It gives birth to impulses within us that can be very strong, as in Talia's case – it caused her desire to heal her mother. In other cases, we might suppress, deny, or sacrifice our own needs, wishes, goals, emotions, etc.

** Who belongs to your original family system?

- You
- Your parents
- Your grandparents
- Your great-grandparents, and so on
- Your siblings
- Your parents' siblings
- Former partners of parents, grandparents, and so on
- Pets

Sometimes even events or other energies, such as secrets, God/religion, war and death, victims and perpetrators, etc. (see list below*)

* Who belongs to your present family system?

- You
- Whoever you have chosen as a partner – present or past
- Their partners
- Their children and your children from before
- Children you have together
- Pets

Sometimes other energies, like work, secrets, religion, abuse, etc. (see list above**)

How does a disturbance in the bonding show? One example might be that you want nothing to do with this person anymore, or you might even deny that you have anything to do with this person. A common consequence is that you don't accept that part of you which comes from them. Sometimes we even destroy what might otherwise be a strength within us because we deny our connection to the person who is its source. You might sabotage your own growth or success, because, in the end, all these parts do belong to you, not only those that you are able to accept. Those parts you don't accept then have so much power over you that they hold you hostage, devaluing yourself in order to continue to deny the original bond. This impacts your decisions, thoughts, actions, which partner you choose, and so on.

- How do you find yourself in relation to these ideas?
- How does that influence your self image and your life in general?

- What would have to happen so that you could accept a little bit more some gifts you might have that come from someone with whom you would rather deny a connection?
- What kind of gifts are they?
- How might embracing these gifts free you?

The balance between giving and receiving within the family system looks at the basic wheel that drives life: children receive life from their parents... and life is one of the biggest gifts you can receive; without it, you wouldn't be there. Also given by the parents are values, food, shelter, protection... and children receive. Usually the children feel the 'imbalance' of so much receiving, and wish to give back. Actually this 'imbalance' is, in this case, a positive, creative force: we need only shift from the thought of giving back to one of giving forward – to their own children (although perhaps some of these basic gifts are given back to the parents, but later in life).

What of this concept between siblings? Going back to the original family, this dynamic is also affected by the birth order. The firstborn had the parents to themselves. So when other siblings are born, a need to share the parents is created. The firstborn has received more, so, to create a balance, there must be more giving. Thus, they are expected to help take care of the younger children. Now there is a balance in the giving and receiving. The same idea applies to the last born. They are often the ones who take care of the parents in old age; this balances all they received from the parents and the older siblings.

Let us look at disturbances in this balance between giving and receiving. If one is receiving more than they are giving, feelings of guilt can arise, often with a desire to give back. Conversely, there might be a relationship where one is giving all the time, and ends up feeling 'used' or that they are being taken advantage of. Extreme examples of imbalances in giving and receiving are those of abuse:

emotional, energetic, verbal, mental, physical, sexual, or spiritual abuse. Family constellation work is effective here too. Often, victims of abuse see themselves as the problem; when we look at the situation in terms of giving and receiving, they can see that in fact, they are giving too much… and the space for healing is open.

- Where do you have to deal with these imbalances in your life?
- If you are feeling 'used' by someone, how would it feel to leave the responsibility for their decision to take too much, with them?
- How would it feel if you took for yourself this freedom: to give yourself the permission to withdraw from certain situations and people, while maintaining the right to love them?
- Is there someone around whom you are feeling guilt? What would happen if you took responsibility for the decisions you made?
- What does that tell you about decisions you would like to make in the future?

Sometimes, we might take on a destiny of our parents or forefathers, and don't realize the impact this has on our lives. This is called entanglement. It is possible to have stepped into this dynamic without being aware of it. See if this is familiar, as it is a common way entanglements manifest: you have discerned a pattern in your life, but you don't understand why you re-engage in it. "I don't understand why I keep picking the wrong partners." "I don't understand why I'm always concerned about money." "I don't understand why I'm always so sad – in truth my life is pretty complete." These are often signs of entanglement, which creates an imbalance in the family constellation. The good news is there is a driving force that makes it understandable, and it can be worked out. The foundation to remember is this: When you carry your own burdens, you grow, even though it might be hard. But if you carry someone else's burden, it brings you down.

- How is it with you?
- Where might you feel overwhelmed or burdened by carrying somebody else's load?
- What would happen if you consciously chose to only carry your own backpack?
- And here, a double check for parents: do you carry the belief that you should carry your children's backpacks because you gave birth or adopted them?
- How would it influence your children if you trusted that they can somehow carry their own backpack – however they decided to do it? Their way might not be your way.

27
The Miracle Of The Group/Family
GROUP CONSCIOUSNESS: MIRACLE OR MAYHEM?

You are somehow always a part of a group. This group builds group consciousness. In this group consciousness, you are connected to the others so that your group can react to outside situations. Originally, this was how the group protected itself, and, as it often happened, served the survival of the species. This remains so today. Together with the group you can fulfill things that you would not be able to do alone.

- What would happen if you took your free will and your self responsibility into the group consciousness
- How would the group consciousness be affected?

In the German book **Vernetzte Intelligenz**, the authors describe very well how we fell from group consciousness into the individual consciousness, which happened about 3,000 years ago. And now we are again coming into a new group consciousness, but with a major difference: now our individuality, our own free will, and our sense of self-responsibility become part of the group consciousness. This raises the energy of the group consciousness in that we no longer create mayhem in our reactions; rather, we make a conscious decision, thus giving birth to an entirely new group consciousness – and the group miracle can take place. So we are stepping out of the either/or reality of the past, and stepping into the 'as-well-as' version… where your individuality is intact and thriving, and by that same token, that serves the enhancement of the group. The days of "there is no "I" in team" are over… now we strengthen "I" to make a stronger "we."

- What do you think?
- How would a strong you strengthen the groups you are part of?
- How would that cycle back, to be part of stronger groups, in supporting a stronger you?

With an eye on individual consciousness, now 'ego' is up for consideration. You can use your inherent ego to give your free will a positive expression. The resulting decisions have more to do with your real life path than the pseudo-decisions our entanglements would make. If you decide out of the positive power of your healthy ego to make your contributions, then you take a starring role in your own movie of Life. By becoming a puzzle piece in the whole grand picture, your inside puzzle pieces come together and you are complete. However, if one acts out of an entangled place instead, although there are still dramatic scenes, you are really in someone else's movie. And you will never get an Oscar for that.

- Are you on an Oscar path? Where in your life can you step more fully into the starring role?
- Standing fully in your free will, what would your movie look like?
- How would you notice that you are acting from the positive power of your healthy ego?

28
The Miracle Of The Group/Family
MAKING HISTORY

Let us now consider the level of existence that transcends space and time from the aspect of all of us that is a piece of a larger whole.

We have focused our discussion so far, primarily, on the whole that is a family. But the ideas here, the basic connections, we know, extend through other groups as well.

- How far does this go, this interplay between the group and the individual?

In truth, it has no limits.

You are part of a family. Likely, at least in your childhood, you were a member of a school. Most of us are members of work groups. We are members of a culture. We are members of a nation. We are members of mankind!

And, just as the web of the family influences us, and is influenced by us, so, too, does the web of each of those groups influence us... and so, too, is it influenced by us.

Physically. Emotionally. Energetically. Mentally. Soul by soul. Person by person.

On the one hand, this can be challenging. Let us take the example of someone who is raised in a culture where it is the mainstream thought that 'progress,' as one grows, takes you through school, to work, to marriage, to owning a house. And let's say you follow that path and find, at some point, that you have done those things, but you don't feel fulfilled.

How can this be?

You followed the prescription. Everyone was doing those things!... they must be 'good' !!!

But still, you don't feel free. You don't feel happy. You don't feel good at all!

Why not?

Perhaps it is because how you would feel happy is not in line with the mainstream – with the group consciousness. Perhaps there is a conflict between your true self expression, and where the culture was at the time you came into it. Perhaps, once you've done your process of self discovery, you find that you feel that it would work better to travel the world, meeting new people. And now, your light goes on.

What happens in that moment? When you step into a place of self understanding? What happens in your body, your emotions, your energy, your mind?

Everything clarifies. Everything brightens. Everything strengthens. You, now in inner alignment, radiate a clearer, sharper energy. Your DNA transmissions are stronger, more powerful, supercharged. Your entire energetic field transmits a different vibe, and attracts that which is like it.

And that affects the energy field – and fields – around you. Just as Talia's mother's behavior changed when Talia clarified her own feelings, so do you become a source of other people stepping into their own alignment. In effect, you become a center of strength that helps others around you gain their own strength. Others in your family. Others in your work group. Others…

How far can this go?
I will tell you. Even national history affects the current generation's consciousness. I will tell you a personal story as an example.

I was born in the USSR. My family, in the 1920s, had lost their land and property during the time of Stalin, and had been removed to labor camps. When I came to Germany later, I could see there was a very heavy energy of guilt and blame around Hitler and World Wars I and II. But I had not felt this in Russia! I was researching why this was so. Having a British husband, I had the opportunity to talk to English people about the Commonwealth, about India and the Aborigines of Australia. Their energy was different too! I was also traveling a lot, and talked to the Americans as well – and their attitude was different too! I couldn't understand it. Why is that, that one nation kills people and feels burdened, and another nation kills people and doesn't?

My research confirmed that there is, indeed, great difference in the later generations' consciousness depending on whether a nation won or lost a war.

We know that within the family system, the past affects the present. Yes. Why should it be different with a nation?

The energy system is still self balancing – still the net of which we are but one eye, but ever connected to the whole. To all of space, to all of time. Intentions are the force that drives creation… if our ancestors sought to expand themselves, and acted that out through war, and then lost… that unmet intention will have an effect on today. Were it not for the fact that we know WE can also affect the whole, this might be very very heavy.

But we can affect the whole.

In my research, I came across the physical anchor point for this energetic dynamic. It has been found that history itself is imprinted in our DNA in the form of miasmas. A miasma is coded information within our gene molecule that derives from the stories of our forefathers – for instance, if someone's ancestors experienced the unmet intention of self expansion (as in the wars), the generations that follow come in imprinted with that code. Now in Germany we see expansion in many cultural expressions – including the broadened understandings of how life works brought through in Bert Hellinger's family constellation work!

So even things from the past can affect us. And still, we have the tools, the guidance, and the direction to turn our light on. And still, when we do, the energy of the whole is affected by us.

The message actually is that when you are aware that something is unfinished because you discern a difference between your conscience and the group conscience, instead of pointing the finger, it's good to use the energy, to be aware of this that we described, and to tidy up the history, your own system. To allow the truth is spoken out. To create a new order which will can be installed in the whole, creating a place from which the group, be it family or nation can move on. That's the message. There is a happy end.

The underlying message is this: YOU COUNT. If you ever thought, "I can't change history, I can't do anything about what's going on in the world," that's not true. You're a ripple in the pond. You can't change history but you can change how it is written in the present. You can change the energetic field NOW, and it will have a domino effect on the past and the future. Like it has a domino effect within the family, so too, the world. It's not about being better or worse than someone else, it's about the fact that you count. I had a lot of patients who had ancestors who were very influential on world politics, and they were still suffering from things that were not put in the right dynamic and order. It doesn't matter whether it was in Hawai'i, in Germany, in America, they all reacted the same. When we did systemic healing, they all felt the relief of sometimes centuries of burdens falling off them.

YOU COUNT.

You count. Suppose you could accept that you count a little bit:

What would you like to do next?
- For yourself?
- Your family?
- Your ancestors?
- Your country?

How would that influence
- You?
- Your family?
- Your ancestors?
- Your country?
- The world in general?

What do you think?

29
No Miracles Without Soul
LOOK WHO'S TALKING

What does 'soul' mean for you?

'Thinking' about the soul, I get into contact with eternity. With infinity and the awareness of Pure Being. I become some sort of idea that I am not this flesh and blood, but that I use my flesh and blood as an instrument – as a home, or even as a playground – in order to make human experiences.

- Who is it that is having these experiences?
- Who is it that is aware?

The soul. I perceive her like a sun. Yes! Like a sun! Deep inside there is the soul nucleus, and outside the streams of light, which beam out in my interactions with my environment. The nucleus of the soul is pure, untouchable, and enlightened. The streams have the task of making experiences which make it clear to me that this radiant nucleus exists inside me. The streams make the experience of how it is when I am separated, and how it is to feel hurt. That way the soul nucleus and the streams experience what being a Pure Being looks like and what it is that disconnects me from that.

While I am writing about the soul I realize that I am getting calmer and calmer. Feelings of security and peace unfold deep inside me. While I am using these words to describe this, I realize that there is nothing that can describe it. This awareness is too big, too deep, too wide, too clear, to ever fit inside any word. It is as if I tried to put the whole universe into a small little vessel and nevertheless I feel this universe in its miniature in every single cell.

Your soul shows you in many ways if you are on the right path.

- Is that true for you?

- If yes, how does she do that?

OK. To be honest, the rest of your 'stuff' - your body, mind, emotions, etc. – they might not agree with your soul. But you can count 100% on your soul.

- When have you had this experience?

She – your soul – is the wisest teacher. She is the answer to all your questions. She is the miracle that you tried to find somewhere outside, in vain. She was there before you had this body and she will still be there when you leave it. An energy which personifies the awareness without being a person.

- What do you think about the soul?

The soul is an energy that doesn't care what you think about her. She will never give herself up only because you give yourself up. !! Wow! What kind of security is that?

Aaah. By the way... who is it that is reading this?
- Hmmm.

What is it that is talking to you here?
- Hmmm.

What else is our soul?
Parmahansa Yogananda, a powerful spiritual teacher, once said, "Stillness and movement as one. Stillness in the movement and movement in the stillness."

- How do you experience that?

She is more patient than the rest of me is... which may not be a big deal, because I am, in general, impatient. And she is also an artist who creates and destroys – without being self-impressed.

Which part of me is aware of that?
- Hmmm.

Do you know what I am talking about here? Which part of you knows?
- Hmmm.

So what is the soul for you, finally?
For me, it is the soul nucleus – it is like a smiley, knowing and loving, seeing through all my little plans while I wind myself up with nothingness... and it stays patient, and stays with me. Until I am done. It smiles at me without laughing at me. It carries all my judgment without being affected by them. It shows me how fleeting everything is that's not her.

What is left when everything you held onto so tightly is gone? It is the soul.

30
No Miracles Without Soul
THE CAMEL MAY NOT HAVE GONE THROUGH THE EYE OF THE NEEDLE YET…

- What is a miracle on the soul level for you?
- What does that mean for you?

For me, it means, to live one's true potential. To fulfill your soul purpose and to take your place in the big picture. Let's say we were born with individual talents in order to use them for the highest good of everybody. Not to use them would cause atrophy in those talent 'muscles.' The inner soul nucleus wouldn't be bothered by that, but the streams of light reaching out might be affected. Those streams are the parts that interact with other realities, with other soul streams, which might also react to you not using your own talents as well. This is why issues on the soul level can manifest even though the soul nucleus stays healthy.

In this case, you might not feel well in your body anymore. Or you might even disconnect from certain soul parts of you. You may even experience a longing to go back 'home.' And sometimes, the space that should be filled with you, with all your soul parts, gets filled with others' energy. Then you might not even feel like yourself anymore... like someone else is in the drivers' seat. Apathetic. Lifeless. Dull.

- When did you experience something like that?
- How did you get out of it again?

All these things could be a sign that something is not quite right on the soul level. Of course, there can be other root causes for that, like physical, systemic, mental, or emotional-energetic challenges. But what happens when it happens on the soul level?

You stop experiencing yourself as a spark of the divine. You're disconnected from yourself and you try to fill this inner emptiness with something artificial – like TV, eating, drinking, or other habits. Your life might not feel fulfilled anymore, and is colored by inactivity, negativity, hopelessness and pessimism.

- When do you have experiences like this?
- What triggers you?
- What could you do to prevent that?

You know your life purpose when you and your soul have a familiar relationship. The challenges in your life don't pull you down; rather, they connect you with your purpose. They even connect you with your real soul nucleus.

- When have you experienced this state?
- What would you have to do to have more of these moments?

Finally you realize that the miracle you were looking for

outside, is inside. There unfolds an inner calm... and you relax, totally supported. You lose the urge to react, and choose, instead, when to act. The camel may not yet have gone through the eye of the needle... but you... you'll greet him when he arrives.

The decisions that you make when you are in this heavenly state come directly from the soul nucleus, rather than from the survival instinct or fear or panic anymore. You are carrying a clear, instinctive Knowing within of who you really are, and how you would like to use your time on earth. And you put it into action!

Trust and faith develop out of knowledge, out of your experiences, and finally out of wisdom awareness. They are not illusions, not just in your mind. You become aware of feeling – you Are – a presence and a strength... other people are aware too.

This is the power that penetrates everything. It gives you a feeling of being complete, on all the levels we have described so far. That doesn't mean that we can only heal the soul directly on the soul level... sometimes we address the soul by healing the body, or doing a systemic ritual, or finding an emotional-energetic solution. As we will see later in this book, the level Beyond Time and Space is also connected to the soul level and can provide a space for healing as well.

- What does your soul need to feel completely whole and at peace?
- Where are you, in this process, in your life right now?
- What would you have to do not to change that?

31

No Miracles Without Soul
LIFE PURPOSE: SOUL CHAMPIONSHIP IN THE BODY OLYMPICS

- How do you find your life purpose?
- How might your life benefit from knowing it?
- Suppose you had found it already... what would change for you?

There are many possible ways to find your life purpose. The simplest answer seems to be: follow the inner road - your own longings – to get to Home.

What are you really seeking? Is it freedom? Love? To make a difference in the world? Fame? Creativity? Fortune?

Any answer is okay. Who would judge you? The soul doesn't. Or don't you dare anymore to explore your true longings... and to find them? Did you even somehow lose the connection to your birthright to be who you really are?

Oh! Then you have to change that. Immediately.

And I am sure you can do that.

Because of the endlessness of the soul, she doesn't give us any limitations: "That's not possible! Who do you think you are?" These thoughts come from the field of false programming about who we really are, what we are allowed to do and what we aren't. And we know that the programming of the nervous system began in the womb, and had a major effect on us in the first 6 years of our lives. The good news is that if you were programmed once, you can be programmed again. This is exactly what some scientists, like Bruce Lipton, say... and I share this opinion – because it gives me the feeling of being a creator in the universe, not a victim.

What do you believe?

Let us say you are ready to step out of being identified with, for instance, a seeker. Searching, searching, searching... instead, you make yourself a Finder. You catch yourself finding things. You use the soulbound archetypes in order to be able to do that. A real SoulFinder who creates all these things, in the end doesn't care anymore what kind of soul he or she is... you use All possibilities on the soul level to live the soul purpose, here on the physical plane. So if you are a healer, or a combination of healer and priest, even though you might find yourself in this kind of soulbound archetype, you live the freedom that you also use the warrior qualities, or the king archetype, or the magician archetype,... because on this level, you are beyond needing any identification at all.

Let's go to another aspect of the soul: she creates constantly. Which is a very powerful trait. If you are aware of this, you can take this power in your own hands. If you are not aware of it, it might be that you experience yourself being like the baseball in the game of life, instead of the player... note that on the soul level, the rules are different. This might make you think of yourself as a victim, which is a physical level look at this metaphor... but remember that on the soul level, you are actually player, playing field... and ball.

Nonetheless, because we experience our lives on the physical level, it is important to appreciate that. To remember that this is the very nature of the game our soul is about right now. As such, the physical level is to be honored. Wounds must be addressed and each player made whole on the physical level in order to fully master this game. And, on the physical level, often those wounding scenes are carried out with actors who play victims and actors who play perpetrators.

When you live a challenge on the physical level, like perpetrator and victim, and you address it, you can move out of this dynamic. You can move on.

For example. When you have found yourself having been a victim of any kind of abuse, it is important to name the perpetrator, give them the guilt and responsibility for what they have done. It is important to name the victim and pronounce their innocence in this situation as well, so that they don't carry the consequences anymore, and can move forward in their lives.

Remember how we said the mind was the glimmer that gives the body a soul? One of its tasks is to try to declare our role. Understand that we naturally have a passion for identity and archetype - how you define yourself, how you identify yourself. And in fact, most of us hold a very strong opinion about who we Are, and who we Are Not. This can be helpful! But we must be aware... often the way we define ourselves is very earthbound. I am a wife, I am an Englishman, I am spiritual, I am a woman... Still, this is useful, because when we come in and get these bodies, the drama is so vast, it is helpful to know your role so that some things have to do with you and some things do not.

We further define ourselves in terms of qualities... I am too stupid, I am not worthy, I am a poor person... yes, these are in fact belief systems, not actual Truths... but the languaging, and our repetition of them, can result in our defining ourselves thus.

So. An invitation. How would it be if you were to create new expressions which are more soul bound? Because the soul creates all the time, you can rely on this innate creativity to make ideas that serve on a broader basis. German author Varda Hasselmann describes Archetypes of the Soul in her book artistically and elegantly. (The book is now translated into English.) I just want to give you some examples of the soulbound archetypes:

- The healer
- The king
- The warrior
- The teacher
- The magi (Like the biblical 3 Wise Men)
- The magician

...and so on. How are these archetypes different from our earthbound identification systems? In this life, you might not be a king. But, you might need the qualities and talents of a king to really fulfill what you have chosen as your soul purpose in this life. Connecting to this archetype, then, you can plug in and download the gifts of that archetype in order to help you fulfill what you have chosen on the highest level. Independent of whether you are a king in this life or not! ... mostly, likely, you are not. We just don't have enough kings anymore.

Similarly, as we discussed earlier, when we come to those times in our lives when we find ourselves screaming, "Only a miracle can help me!" - you actually reach out and plug into the archetype of a magician and download magician qualities to open yourself up – even your nervous system – and to close synapses that might not have served you. Then you open up new pathways that weren't necessary before, but which now are essential to really create miracles.

What do you think?

Soul championship in the body Olympics? Or is it a body championship in the soul Olympics?

Which perpetrator/victim dynamic wants to be addressed in your life, on the physical level?

Imagine you have progressed through this dynamic on the physical level… what is waiting there on the soul level?

Sometimes, inviting new ways of thinking of yourself can bring up fear. Remember the old synapses that we talked about? That close up as they are no longer needed? We can think of this as old attachments – even attachments to how we think of ourselves. We don't have to let the old identity die – it was valid and important and it is part of us and the path we have walked. But the attachment to it, if we let that go, can be replaced with a progressive attachment to a new identification. Yes, there is a funeral to attend – but it isn't the funeral of a part of you, just the cord that binds you to it too tightly.

- Which archetype costumes will you wear to the funeral(s)?
- Which cords of attachment that used to tie you in knots now lie in the coffin, making way for the new in your life?

32
No Miracles Without Soul
IN THIS WORLD, BUT NOT OF IT...

We know that every one of us has this brilliant DNA that sends and receives information, continuously, throughout the universal energy field. We have energy centers working together in our chakras; we each have a morphogenetic field that is a system of great power, that is always with us. The universe itself is a morphogenetic field of energy. That means you are an expression of the divine force, that you are connected to the divine creative force, in every moment.

Think of the possibilities. Even psychic abilities are now understood by Garjajev's research. As continuous senders and receivers of light, information, and energy, we have many talents inherent within us that we don't ordinarily use. And you can strengthen these abilities, like training any other muscle. For instance, meditation expands your consciousness and the frequency range of information that you are nimble in perceiving.

You are a soul with a role to play. You are ever connected to the universal field of knowledge and wisdom, and you have a built in receiving mechanism that is attuned to your particular purpose in this lifetime.

Time not a limiter. Not only does this hold true within your own lifetime, but also, as we have seen in earlier sections, beyond (future and past) your lifetime. This means you even have access to learning, gifts, and skills from your past lives!

Old souls and young souls in cooperation (I don't know where you wanted to go with this)

How do you stand strong in this new awareness of yourself and create miracles? On the soul level, often, we pray. Yogananda said praying is talking to God and meditation is listening to God. So when we go into meditation or prayer, we open up to receive answers to the soul's questions.

Yogananda taught that, to pray powerfully, to pray from this truth, we should pray not from a beggar's attitude, but instead as if we are knocking on heaven's door with persistence. Remembering that we are already connected to the source of creation which, by definition, is where all that we would like, is created. Using that grateful awareness that we talked about earlier to joyfully participate in the creation of our wishes, with clear visions, strong feelings, aligned intentions, and powerful words. Remembering that we even have a connection to that which we are praying for.

Sometimes we have the feeling that our prayers are not heard. Sometimes unsolved ego issues might come in and think they know what's best for our souls. I submit: they might not be right. The lower ego may have an idea what it would look like, to receive what you asked for, or to be guided. Here your soul steps in. When you know it's just the lower aspect of the ego and not the rest of you, you choose to trust that that which is on your soul's brightest path will manifest; you just smile about the egoic versions and receive your messages, guidance, and fulfillment in a totally different way.

When there are soul-level contracts, vows or promises

from other lives still active now, such as a monk's vows of poverty or celibacy, this can prevent you from stepping into your soul purpose in this life as well. Again, I don't want you to just believe this – if this part doesn't ring true with you, forget it. But if you feel blocked, you might want to consider whether something is hanging on from the past that is not aligned with Now. As if you are taking your final exams in high school, you wouldn't use the books from first grade! Here, it serves to recalibrate yourself on this level as well so you give your system totally different commands that are appropriate for this life and this life's purpose.

Remember, intention counts.

33

Outside Of Time And Space
COMMUNICATING WITH THE WHALES

This is a story that I like to share in my DNA Reformatting seminars and I wish to share with you now. First I want to focus a moment on the DNA itself. It is, as you probably know, the deoxyribo nucleic acid, our gene molecule. But there's so much more than we were first taught… More on that to come…

- Do you know the power place of your soul?
- Would you like to know it?
- How could you find out?

I was lucky enough to know the power place of my soul, and I am very very grateful for it. It is the island of Kaua'i, one of the chain of Hawaiian islands. When I am there, I am always open. This was the state of affairs when this story took place.

My husband Paul and I were on a whale watching excursion. No, we had booked a trip to swim with dolphins. But I had a longing inside me to see the whales.

Ever since I was small, I felt a very deep connection to these ocean wanderers, without having known what was behind it. Somehow I always know where they are and where to look to find them. But why? I have no clue.

On this trip, something very exceptional happened. This connection to the whales somehow guided us to a whole big group of whales, a whole bunch, and we were in the middle of it. They were jumping beside the boat, jumping very high. My husband was very afraid in fact! And all I thought was, "this is it." This was what I had experienced in meditation... and now it was there, in real life. I had no fear at all... it was just being home. And I knew they were making a present to us – to all of us who were in this boat. I was very grateful for this deep connection because I knew it was part of the reason we were allowed to come together like this. And again, it was a soul experience because I just felt safe, grateful, and even though my mind didn't understand half of what was going on, after the experience, things happened in my body that were life changing, because of this experience with the whales. I was told by the Hawaiians that whales have the potential to change one's DNA. But at that point in my life I had no clue how important this information would be only 2 years later.

Two years later. I was in this state of mind between sleeping and awake, back in Hawai'i. And I observed myself sitting up and screaming, "Now I know!!" ... and my own screaming woke me up. But somehow even though I was awake then, I could remember where I was while I was doing that. I was in a place where I was connected with the whales, and for the first time in my life it was conscious. I was aware. I could feel that my whole body – every cell – inside every cell – there was like a reorganization going on. They were vibrating inside and coming into a new order. And while I was still feeling this, in my body, my mind started to understand that my DNA was in a process of reprogramming. And I somehow knew that I had to find additional information which explains this process that happened inside me. So I stood up, and usually I don't know how to deal with the computer at all... but I was standing up, guided by a force that was big, big, big... and I was going to the computer, and I found myself finding the right information in the computer which was out of the book I referred to before, the vernetzte intelligenz. I found something about that on the internet... or it found me. So I was doing research – actually, it was half reading all the stuff, still having this process in the cells going on, it was like downloading right into my body, speed reading, and somehow, this came from the mind and at the same time the body process was still going on and it came together like WHOOSH! I was going to the beach then still in this WHOOSH, and I saw the whales jumping again. I knew this was the confirmation that this was the information I needed and I was to bring it forth. What kind of information was that? Scientific information from Garjajev and his team, and the spiritual knowledge that the whales helped me to remember. And I just Knew, all of a sudden, after groping in the dark for two years, so clearly what was happening to me. Which I already said when I was waking up, but I didn't understand why I was saying that... and now I understood.

It was about bringing it together and presenting it, in workshops and meditation, so that everybody can have access to it.

But why am I really telling you this?

It has a lot to do with our DNA. And its task which is described as being the birthplace for any communication, beyond time and space. Garjajev found out that 90% of the so-called 'silent' DNA is actually quite the opposite of what you would think... it's the birthplace for every kind of communication, like nonverbal communication and exchange of information on all kinds of levels. It has the capacity to attract and to save information, and to send out information. It has the ability to emit light, which explains why enlightened people truly radiate light. It has the potential to build wormholes and to close them to facilitate the attracting and receiving of information. And it has the ability to create spontaneous healing to restructure itself… and to be influenced by our thoughts, words, deeds, environment, and experiences. It is the playground for what we call 'intuition.' And now I begin to understand how the whales and I are interacting. We are communicating on a nonverbal level.

- When did you experience something that hints at your ability to communicate nonverbally?
- Is there a place you feel, think about, are drawn to, even if you have never been there? What would you find about yourself if you were to go there?
- What about plants, stones, other people… no matter where they are?
- How would you like to use your inherent ability to communicate nonverbally? To give your role as SoulFinder even more power?
- When did you experience something that you could only explain as, "I just Know."?
- And how would you explain experiences like that, now that you know these things about your DNA?

In fact, in essence, in truth… as everything that we perceive, and all that we are, is energy, then miracles are, in actuality, everywhere… every moment… everyone.

34
The Last Words
CONCLUSION

What conclusions do you draw from this book – from your own journey:

- For yourself?
- For your health?
- For your relationships?
- For your life?
- For your vocation?
- For your soul?
- In any other areas?

I want to share with you what I experienced while I was writing this book. It was very important for me, this process of writing. I rediscovered, by doing this, a part of me that I thought I had lost. And I hadn't even remembered anymore. It is the Rita that I was when I was three years old. Courageous. Determined. She never hid, no matter what. As a three-year-old, I once decided to pick up my father from his job, on my tricycle. Determined as I was, I didn't care that I had to drive over a big road with lots of traffic, I had to pass a great big German Shepherd (that I was afraid of), and, that there was a security door at his workplace that required a secret combination to be punched in to enter. For a three year old girl, obstacles like that were big! But in that time, I never doubted for a second that I could do it. My decision, Now I will pick Papa up at work, was all. Now that I had started, nothing would stop me. I know that I thought, "Eh, you can do this somehow…"

So I was pedaling along. I knew how to cross the road somehow, when I got there. The dog? Wasn't even there. And the secret code? No problem – I once watched my father typing it in, just a few weeks before, and I decided, "I'll remember that. Never know when I might need it."

So there I was. I didn't see my father. The next person who crossed my path asked,

"What are you doing here?"

"I'm picking up my Papa!"

"Who is your Papa?"

So I gave him the name, and he did the rest of my work for me. When Papa showed up, he was really proud of me. He picked me up and introduced me to his colleagues. He was really, really proud.

And I was proud of myself!

Then something happened when I came home … my mother was not so proud. ;) She really was shocked that I did that. As you can imagine. So she punished me, according to the pain I caused inside her. And I must admit this punishment affected me. I replaced my feeling of courage with self doubt. And the rest of the story is like being trapped in some sort of nightmare. I really would say that.

But now! It's time to wake up! Something happened! I am waking from the nightmare! I am awake. I am here. I hope that I can pick you up on my tricycle as well.

Have fun riding your own tricycle.

ABOUT THE AUTHOR

If you feel hindered by trauma; family of origin issues; physical or emotional pain or fatigue; if you want to feel lighter, freer, more authentic and more powerful; if your life is good and you're ready for it to be great - I urge you, come and meet Rita...
Mary McDonald Lewis
Screen Actors Guild

Rita is one of the best coaches I have ever observed at work. She has a natural ability to zoom in on the issues at the core and to bring clients to fast insight. I recommend her highly for profound, guided work. Dr.
Dr. Hiyaguha Cohen Ph.D.
Life-Change Coach

Rita has helped me uncover, understand and help the real me in a manner that is unique, fast and powerful. She has podcasts, group and personal sessions at her place of business in Long Beach or via Facetime. I cannot say enough about this woman.
Dana Ouimette
Tax Professional

I have experienced first hand the depth of Rita's healing work. Love yourself, you deserve it. I have faith that you will feel differently after spending time with Rita.
Myriam Haynal

Rita is the founder and practitioner of the Willow System healing modality and has assisted many individuals in the community through private practice, workshops, and seminars in Hawaii and internationally. She has had profound results through the Willow System methods and has trained other professionals in the community, who are interested in promoting optimum health and helping others suffering from psychological and physical pain. She is a consummate professional and I would recommend her to others without reservation.
Ann Dorado
Counselor

Rita is a multi-faceted holistic health professional with techniques addressing the physiological, mental, emotional and spiritual components necessary for healing. She has developed the Willow System out of her many studies and years of practice and I highly recommend her work!
Joan Levy
Clinical Social Worker

The love Rita brings to a therapeutic relationship creates a healing atmosphere which, through the skillful use of kinesiology combined with a highly developed intuition, allows for a return to wholeness within the individual.
Richard Diamond
Blogger

Rita creates a safe place for you to heal the hurt, the pain of today, yesterday and all of your past and that of your ancestors. So you can go forward with a clear heart full of love.
Char Ravelo
Publisher

www.ingramcontent.com/pod-product-compliance
Lightning Source LLC
Chambersburg PA
CBHW031419210526
45464CB00005B/1967